Health and Modernity

The Role of Theory in Health Promotion

Health and Modernity
The Role of Theory in Health Promotion

David V. McQueen
Centers for Disease Control and Prevention
Atlanta, Georgia

and

Ilona Kickbusch
Swiss Federal Office for Health
Bern, Switzerland

With

Louise Potvin
Université de Montreal
Montreal, Canada

Jürgen M. Pelikan
University of Vienna
Vienna, Austria

Laura Balbo
University of Ferrara
Ferrara, Italy

Thomas Abel
Department of Social and Preventive Medicine
University of Bern
Bern, Switzerland

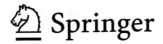 Springer

David V. McQueen
Prevention and Health Promotion
Centers for Disease Control and Prevention
Atlanta, Georgia 30341
USA

Ilona Kickbusch
Swiss Federal Office for Health
Bern 3013
Switzerland

Library of Congress Control Number: 2006932835

ISBN 10: 0-387-37757-3   e-ISBN-10: 0-387-37759-X
ISBN 13: 978-0-387-37757-5   e-ISBN-13: 978-0-387-37759-9

Printed on acid-free paper.

9 8 7 6 5 4 3 2 1

springer.com

Acknowledgments

As will be apparent to even the most casual reader, this book took considerable time to produce and was the fruit of many discussions, exciting and tedious, but always with a tone that the authors wanted to really understand the theory behind their thinking. In many ways it was a luxury that few working in health promotion have, that is, to take the time to engage in the discourse that is needed to more fully understand one's point of view. If the end product is not the quintessential theory of health promotion, it is not the fault of those organizations and individuals about to be acknowledged.

Among the organizations to be thanked are those affiliated with two of the authors, Louise Potvin, at the University of Montreal and Thomas Abel, Department of Social and Preventive Medicine at the University of Bern, Switzerland. These organizations provided wonderful settings for comprehensive face-to-face meetings. Special thanks for ongoing support go to the Health Promotion Switzerland in Bern and the National Center for Chronic Disease Prevention and Health Promotion at the Centers for Disease Control and Prevention (CDC), Atlanta. Both organizations provided most appropriate settings for open discussions of the content of the book, as well as resources, space, and time for editing and analysis of the prepared chapters by the authors.

Two individuals in Atlanta worked diligently on the development and completion of the book: Mary Hall for assisting in the early days of the book and for keeping track of the agreements among the authors on how to proceed; and in the later stages of the book's development Andrea Neiman was a champion for reading all the texts carefully and editing the prose of the five authors for whom English is not their first language. Both of these young women are talented beyond their years, and the authors are most appreciative of their help in making sometimes difficult theoretical abstractions more understandable.

Atlanta, Georgia   David V. McQueen
Bern, Switzerland   Ilona Kickbusch

Contents

Contributors

David V. McQueen is a Senior Biomedical Research Scientist and Associate Director for Global Health Promotion at the National Center for Chronic Disease Prevention and Health Promotion (NCCDPHP), at the Centers for Disease Control and Prevention (CDC) in Atlanta, Georgia, USA. Prior to joining the Office of the Director, he was Director of the Division of Adult and Community Health at NCCDPHP and Acting Director of the Office of Surveillance and Analysis at NCCDPHP. Before joining CDC, he was Professor and Director of the Research Unit in Health and Behavioral Change at the University of Edinburgh, Scotland (1983–1992), and prior to that Associate Professor of Behavioral Sciences at the Johns Hopkins University School of Hygiene and Public Health in Baltimore. He has served as Director of the World Health Organization (WHO) Collaborating Centers as well as a technical consultant with the World Bank. Academic training: MA in History and Philosophy of Science (Johns Hopkins), Doctorate in Behavioral Sciences, Medical Sociology (Johns Hopkins).

Ilona Kickbusch is now a private health consultant and was formerly Head of the Division of Global Health at Yale University School of Medicine in the Department of Epidemiology and Public Health. She joined Yale after a long career with the World Health Organization where she initiated the Ottawa Charter for Health Promotion and headed a range of innovative programs. She has published widely on the new public health and is the founder and chair of the editorial board of the journal *Health Promotion International*. Honors and awards for her achievements include the Andrija Stampar Medal from the Association of Schools of Public Health in the European Region, the meritorious gold medal of the City of Vienna and the Salomon Neumann Medal of the German Society for Social Medicine. She continues to act as an advisor to the World Health Organization and the Pan American Health Organization and a range of foundations, NGOs, and the private sector on matters of global health and the development of health promotion. Presently she acts as the senior health advisor to the United Nations Association of the USA's global health campaign. She has also been designated the distinguished Fulbright New Century Scholars Leader on "Challenges of Health in a Borderless

World." She received her Ph.D. in political science at the University of Konstanz, Germany.

Louise Potvin has a doctorate in Public Health. She is professor at the Department of Social and Preventive Medicine, Université de Montreal and researcher at the Interdisciplinary Health Research Group. She holds the (CHSRF/CIHR) Canadian Health Services Research Foundation/Canadian Institutes of Health Research Chair on Community Approaches and Health Inequalities, which documents how public health interventions in support of local social development contribute to the reduction of health inequalities in urban settings. Her main research interests are the evaluation of community health promotion programs and how local social environments are conducive to health. She was a member of the WHO Working Group on the evaluation of health promotion.

Jürgen M. Pelikan is Professor and Director, Institute for Sociology, University of Vienna; Director, Ludwig Boltzmann-Institute for the Sociology of Health and Medicine; WHO Collaborating Centre for Health Promotion in Hospitals and Healthcare; Former Coordinator of the International Network of Health Promoting Hospitals of WHO-Euro, and is involved in projects of Healthy Cities and Healthy Schools. He has a Dr. Phil. in sociology from the University of Vienna; is trained in psychoanalysis and group dynamics; and is a management trainer and systemic organization consultant. He has been a postdoctoral fellow of the Ford Foundation at Columbia University, New York, a Visiting Scholar at Griffith University, Brisbane, Australia, a former President of the European Society of the Sociology of Health and Medicine, and a consultant with WHO-EURO, WHO-HQ, and the EC. Major research areas: Sociological Systems Theory, Sociology of Organizations, Sociology of Health and Medicine, Public Health and Health Promotion, Health Promotion in Health Care, Health Systems Analysis, Quality Management and Evaluation.

Laura Balbo is Professor of Sociology, University of Ferrara and President of the Italian Sociological Association. She was a member of the Italian Parliament from 1983 to 1992; minister of equal opportunity, 1998–2000; special advisor to the Prime Minister on issues of racism and xenophobia, June 2000–June 2001. Main areas of research: the sociology of higher education and work, the sociology of everyday life, gender studies, racism, and xenophobia. She has been a visiting scholar at the Radcliffe Institute for Independent Studies and at the Center for European Studies at Harvard, and a visiting Associate Professor at the University of California, Santa Cruz. She has also been a consultant with WHO, Copenhagen, with UNESCO, and presently with various committees and study groups of the European Commission.

Thomas Abel is Professor for Health Research at the Institute of Social and Preventive Medicine at the University of Bern, Switzerland. He is also Co-Editor-in-Chief of Social and Preventive Medicine, International Journal of Public Health. Prior to his appointment in Bern, he was Professor for Public Health and Epidemiology, Postgraduate Program in Public Health, Department of Medicine at the Ludwig-Maximilians-University in Munich, Germany (1993–1995); Research Assistant and Lecturer in Medical Sociology, Department of Medicine at the Philipps-University in Marburg, Germany (1986–1993); as well as Teaching and Research Assistant, Department of Sociology at the University of Illinois, Urbana-Champaign, USA (1984–1986). He has served as reviewer and consultant for major national and international research institutions and funding agencies. Academic training: Prior to his habilitation at the Philipps-University (Department of Medicine, 1993), Thomas Abel received his Ph.D. from the University of Illinois (Department of Sociology) in 1989, a Dr. Phil. degree from the Justus Liebig-University (Department of Sports Science) in 1984, and his M.A. degree there in 1980.

1
Introduction

Health Promotion: The Origins of the Third Public Health Revolution Leading to a New Public Health

DAVID V. MCQUEEN* AND ILONA KICKBUSCH

1. Why a Book on Theory and Health Promotion?

Health promotion has long sought to define itself, and this has been an admirable, if futile, pursuit. It is not that there have been unsatisfactory definitions put forward over the years; it is, rather, that on careful scrutiny most fall short of describing the essence of health promotion as a field of study and practice. Most people in the field recognize the comprehensive nature of health promotion and the broad base of it practice. This, in turn, makes any short or simple definition seemingly impossible. Perhaps the field cannot be defined but left open to extensive explanations of its practice. Nonetheless, the seeming inability to clearly define the dimensions of such a major endeavor leaves many, and particularly the authors of this book, with a sense of frustration. As with most frustrations, one seeks to get to the underlying reasons for the difficulties and that is when one asks "deeper" questions about the origins and meaning of the field. That is why the two chief protagonists of this book (Kickbusch & McQueen) searched for solace in theory.

Theory is almost always seen as an abstruse topic and many seek to avoid it. But theory is also the ultimate source for understanding the nature of things. It stems from the quest to develop a philosophy of understanding. Some people are not troubled by trying to grasp deeper meanings, but others are deeply troubled by simple answers. This book is written by those who are somewhat obsessed with understanding the meaning of health promotion and not by those who are content to just practice what they believe.

Thus the rationale for this book is rather straightforward: It is an effort to try to reach a critical understanding of what is an appropriate theoretical basis for current health promotion. However, it is not a historical rehashing of how health promotion got to the place that it now occupies in modern society. Rather, it is an effort to show how social theories have led to a society that in its modernity embraces the underlying nature of health promotion. It is, in the main, an effort to show what

---

* The findings and conclusions in the report are those of the author(s) and do not necessarily reflect the views of the Centers for Disease Control and Prevention.

socio-behavioral theories that rely on the individual as the source of action are wanting when explaining the full richness and importance of health promotion.

A second rationale for the book was apparent from the beginning of our work. The six authors were concerned with the lack of representation of social theories in the extant literature on health promotion. There was an underlying belief that there were important social theories in health promotion, but they had been unappreciated by those in the field or, in many cases, unarticulated. There was consternation that a field concerned with the social, the political, the cultural, with context, with groups, with movements, should have fashioned itself as so heavily rooted in the individually-based behavioral theories of health education and psychology. A clear goal was to broaden this narrow perspective.

Six authors working together over a considerable length of time, concentrating and debating aspects of social theory and its application to health promotion does result in a different kind of product. Of course each author concentrates on a perspective that represents their unique theoretical background, however it is fair to say that each author, not only gained from the process of making this book, but also gained new theoretical perspectives. It has been this process that has made this a different kind of theory book. Chapter Two (Potvin & Balbo) discusses the background of the book in some detail. It is our contention that the book as a whole is better understood if the reader has more information about the process of its making. It is part of our effort to be reflexive. What makes this publication unique is that it is neither the theoretical perspectives of six separate individuals nor that of six individuals speaking as one. Rather it is a unique combination of six voices that have listened, debated and incorporated different theoretical ideas. That is not to say that minds were profoundly changed, but they were certainly altered. This is not a trivial consideration because theory heretofore has generally been the product of a single mind. Notably in the social sciences, theory has not been the product of any participatory, explicitly reflexive effort. The field of health promotion, as a type of social science, has been no exception to this assertion. The mere fact that what started out as a book to provide a social science theory for health promotion has morphed into something larger, dealing with concepts of modernity, complexity, cultural capital, communications and systems theories. This was not just an experience in understanding, it was an experience in participation and learning—and was thus an experience that embodied principles and concepts articulated in the field of health promotion.

2. Why Should Practitioners Be Interested in This Book?

It has often been said that there is nothing as practical as a good theory, a phrase attributed to Kurt Lewin (1951) and as a statement it reflects our views. During our public health careers most of us have been involved in work that is applied and often carried out with a heavy emphasis on how we are going to carry out an intervention. In fact, considerable time is often devoted to the nuts and bolts of a project, for example, how to conduct a survey, how to interview, how to engage the community and so on. In the excitement of the day to day challenges one often has little time to examine the theoretical underpinnings of a project, let alone go into a deeper reflexive discourse on why one is doing it. This emphasis on "doing" has its limitations, most prominently that projects will be unexamined and under-evaluated. However, even more profoundly, the emphasis on "doing" has resulted in a dearth of theoretical thinking.

Recently Alexander Rothman (2004) made the case that theory is not simply important as a starting point for interventions, but also that interventions are needed to test and refine theory. Among other points, he argues that "health behavior theories provide an explicit statement of the structural and psychological processes that are hypothesized to regulate behavior" (p. 2). Thus theories contribute directly to questions of intervention effectiveness and ultimately evaluation. Rothman limits his discussion chiefly to behavioral theories of individual change, but the points are equally relevant to social science theory and health promotion interventions in general. We would extend these notions to the role of theory at all stages in the research and practice of health promotion.

When we think about the nature of health promotion practice, particularly its diverse applications on policy, communities, settings, populations and individuals, it becomes apparent that a broad theoretical literature is relevant. Often one is driven at first to look at theories of change, and this has largely been the case in health education, but it is clear to us that theories of context and state are equally important. Social theory has always grappled as much with why there is stability and order as with why there is disorganizationand conflict. Certainly every practical health promotion intervention should examine the whole spectrum of relevant social theory.

Finally, we would argue that health promotion practice has always possessed theoretical underpinnings, just not explicit. That is, there is always an underlying epistemology behind actions even when they are not explicitly stated, even when they are not fully understood by the practitioner, and even where the practitioner would state that they operate with no theoretical base. This book is also about the examination of that implicit and/or explicit theoretical base and more importantly the authors of this book are engaged in the illumination and transformation of that epistemological base.

3. Omissions and What Is Not in the Book

There is no recognized fundamental grand theory of, for or in health promotion. This book does not purport to provide any such grand theory. It is not that the authors would not have enjoyed developing such a theory, but that early on in our discourse the folly of such a grand theory was recognized. Instead we would argue that there are many theoretical sources that are vital for health promotion, and that many excellent sources have been ignored. In our chapters we introduce theoretical sources and theoretical ideas that we believe to be crucially important for health promotion. But it is not an exhaustive list. For those readers who would argue that some important social theoretical position or theory should have been included, we plead mea culpa. However, we challenge those readers to develop those important theoretical ideas for health promotion. We have little fear that the field of health promotion will be overwhelmed by too much theoretical discourse.

Many readers of this book, most notably those who have approached health promotion from a health education background, will be struck by the omission of rationale choice theories. This is purposive. Such theories have considerable merit, but in our view, they have been afforded considerable place in health promotion theoretical thinking and have been well articulated by many others and therefore, we have nothing to add to this perspective. Our concern is with the critical missing perspectives.

Finally, more an apology than an omission, we recognize the limits of our perspectives that are rooted in our Western culture. We trust that our friends and colleagues who have been spared a Western education will view our work with some deference and realization of our limitations. We also recognize our limitations to the Italic and Germanic portions of the Indo-European language family. Thus our epistemological underpinnings are overwhelmingly influenced by literature in this heritage and we would make no claims of universalism with respect to our theoretical explanations.

4. Two Central Assertions or Assumptions of the Authors

The first is that health promotion is the avant-garde of public health. It is the basis of the shift away from the focus of public health on disease to a focus on health. Control and treatment of disease will continue to be paramount, but the challenges of the modern world revolve around creating and maintaining healthy populations. The compression of morbidity and the reduction of burden in an aging, highly populated world will be the driving force behind a focus on health. The second is that health itself is a force for social change. In recent Canadian elections, health was the number one issue; in many other countries it is a dominant part of the political discourse because of the economic consequences, whether the costs are borne by government, private sector or both. Thus health is fundamental to the social fabric of the modern world.

5. How to Read This Book

It is fashionable now to read selected parts and chapters of books. Perhaps this is a result of our busy schedules, perhaps because we often access parts of books and reports off the internet and read these disembodied pieces as if they were meant to stand alone. We hope that the reader will take a holistic approach. Because this book was the product of many discussions, much discourse and lengthy discussion between and among the six authors it has a particular wholeness. It could be taken as a challenge to the reader to discover who was influenced by whom in the ensuing chapters. Three authors in their chapters (Potvin, Abel, and Pelikan) take, more or less, a particular social theoretical stance and apply it in depth to modernity and health promotion. These are exemplary of a more classical approach to writing theory, in that the perspective of a leading social theorist is explored and applied to the field of health promotion. We agree that there should be considerably more of this classical academic approach using other social theorists as exemplars. Nonetheless, the three authors were constantly challenged to justify their points by the group and this lead, in our opinion, to an even sharper analysis of their positions. The other three authors (Balbo, Kickbusch, and McQueen) are more eclectic and synthetic in their approach, but they too were influenced by the "classical" approach. As a result, this is not the theory book that we intended to write, but it is a more approachable book and one that should be read as a whole.

6. Why No Conclusion

Some readers may ask why this book has no concluding chapter. Such a chapter was discussed at length by the authors. It was felt that a conclusion was not empowering, that it somehow was not quite in the spirit of the book nor of health promotion. Instead, we felt that the readers, if they managed to struggle through the entirely, should draw there own conclusions. Secondly, we felt that the discussion was not over, that drawing conclusions would, in fact, bring about a sense that the meal was "fully cooked". With full apologies to Claude Levi-Strauss, we soon realized that we were still in the developmental stages of preparing a socio-theoretical basis for health promotion in the modern world. The three chapters (Potvin, Pelikan and Abel) that take a theoretical idea, derived from social theory, and explore its utility for health promotion illustrate for others how heuristic this effort is.

Our only, tentative conclusion is that the making of a theoretical perspective is a most challenging endeavor. But it is an undertaking that is exciting and worthwhile. The pity is that there is not more time in our busy lives to take the time to reflect on theory, reflect on modernity, and in general think a lot more before acting.

References

Lewin, K. (1951). *Field theory in social science: Selected theoretical papers.* New York, NY: Harper & Row, p. 169.

Rothman, A. J. (2004). Is there nothing more practical than a good theory? Why innovations and advances in health behavior change will arise if interventions are used to test and refine theory. *International Journal of Behavioral Nutrition and Physical Activity, 1,* 1–11.

2
From a Theory Group to a Theory Book

Louise Potvin and Laura Balbo

1. Introduction

The writing of this book started as a project McQueen and Kickbusch had contemplated for a long period before bringing it into reality. As key players for the elaboration of the Ottawa Charter and for the integration of health promotion into major public health institutions (respectively, the US Centers for Disease Control and the World Health Organisation) they were both acutely aware of the need for health promotion to go back to its original theoretical underpinnings rooted in the social sciences for it to fully play its role as a driving force behind a third revolution of public health.

Rooted in Kickbusch's fondness of Bateson's idea that a small group of people meeting regularly for discussing work in progress can produce innovative knowledge; the book's initiators invited a small group of people to join them in the quest to elaborate a bridge and initiate a renewed dialogue between health promotion and the social sciences. A second line of reasoning emerged as being of great relevance to the project; the feeling that people in the social sciences did not appear to be fully aware of the fact that issues of health, wellness, well-being and care-taking are central in the functioning and evolution of modern societies. Such issues do not form one of the many specialized subfields in the different disciplinary contexts. Both in people's everyday life and in policy-making, what we call in this book the *production of health* (in the public as well as in the private sectors, by market and welfare mechanisms as well as personal arrangements) has come to be of primary concern in terms of financing, governance, organizational patterns, and day-to-day strategies.

Discussing their original project during our fifth meeting, McQueen and Kickbusch came up with the following criteria for selecting the group of collaborators to work with them on the book: a broad background in "social something" and a practice in public health writ large; people who were thinkers in their own field but not theoreticians per se; fluency in English; capacity to learn and grow from the process; and "bon vivant" since it was felt that the original two people were difficult enough they did not want to bring extra difficulties. Also, neither Kickbusch nor McQueen wanted true believers of health promotion. In order to progress and tackle the challenges that lay ahead, their intuition was that the field needed critical assessments of its roots, discourse and practice. Finally, they wanted people willing to take a risk. Writing a book is always risky, making it a collective enterprise such as this was much riskier: at any time in the process there was at least one of us who could not figure out where all this was leading to, how we would get there and whether each of us, including oneself, could deliver a piece that would positively contribute to our own discussion and to the advancement of health promotion.

The enterprise of regular face-to-face meetings, bringing scholars from five different countries seems to be a bit old fashion in the age of e-mail and e-writing where interacting monologues are elaborated and pasted together. This chapter is an attempt to share with you, the reader, a bit of the excitement, anxiety and joy that we all experienced in the four years that has elapsed between the first and 7th meeting of what each of us now refers to as "our theory group". We also believe that the book we are able to offer to your scrutiny owes much to the iterative process described in this chapter.

2. Background: Quest for Theory

Several books have been published over the years addressing the topic of health promotion theory. A majority of these books present a wide array of theoretical discourses as foundations for health promotion. Health promotion practitioners have been provided a menu of theories from which to choose depending upon public health issues (see Glanz, Rimer, & Lewis, 2002). Although as a practical field, it is felt that health promotion needs to be able to borrow from other fields, knowledge which in turn can, be put into practice (McLeroy, Steckler, Simons-Morton, & Goodman, 1993), there is a price to pay of not having its own and unique theoretical basis. One of the main problems in the actual approach to theory for health promotion is the lack of cohesion between the discourse and practice of health promotion. Many contributions to health promotion theory only tangentially relate to what is recognized as one of the field's founding documents, the Ottawa Charter, and its agenda, making the field of health promotion vulnerable to loosing sight of its purpose and specificity. The debate on whether health education and health promotion are distinct, overlapping or complementary practices is an example of this vulnerability.

In contrast with the theoretical contributions of the past 20 years, documents written and circulated by scientists and civil servants involved in the development of the Ottawa Charter, dedicated significant space to discuss the social determinants of health and further raised questions of health inequalities. Reflecting upon the unpublished "Background and Principles" (reproduced here in the book's appendix) or to the "Life-Styles and Health" paper published in 1986 (Kickbusch, 1986), it is striking to realise the extent to which these pieces are relevant to contemporary debates on the social production of health (Frohlich, Corin & Potvin, 2001; Williams, 2003). These early papers clearly positioned health not only as a social issue, but also as a social phenomena, the transformations of which parallels those of our society. It is this kind of analysis that was felt as missing from the published health promotion literature and thus, the main purpose for the book McQueen and Kickbusch had in mind was to initiate a conversation that would align more closely health promotion with contemporary social theory.

In what has now become a traditional process for writing a theory book in health promotion, they started to list issues to be covered in a number of chapters for which the contribution of recognized leaders of the field should be sought, and indeed the content of the book was starting to be shaped into 10 chapters from 10 different authors. We leave to you readers the task of reconstructing for yourself who should have written what. This, according to McQueen and Kickbusch turned out to be somewhat of an unsatisfactory process and the project was redesigned before even the first potential author was contacted. It was felt that to provide the field with innovative and insightful theoretical underpinnings, the process itself of writing about theory should be propitious to theoretical discussions and favourable to innovation.

3. Who We Are

Kickbusch and McQueen handpicked four persons to be part of this experiment; each selecting two. Even though the exact criteria to come up with a balanced group were not spelled out at the beginning, it turned out that our composition could stand as a textbook example of equilibrium. There is of course the very obvious gender balance of three male and three female authors. Less obviously, together we represent three generations of writers; the most senior among us have been contributing to scholarly discussions for close to 40 years whereas the youngest have been around roughly for 20 years, as long indeed as the Ottawa Charter. We leave up to you readers to guess who was picked up by whom.

The apparent geographical diversity of our group is worth a little parenthesis. It is of public knowledge that at the time of the writing of the book three of us were living and working in North America and three in Western Europe. For the record, it should be said that Australian authors were not really considered for reasons of travelling convenience; colleagues from the developing countries, it was felt, were not facing the same dilemmas and challenges than those of primary importance for the discourse to be elaborated in the book. This apparent diversity hides more complicated trajectories. Among the three North American authors, McQueen, has spent an important part of his academic career in the UK, the part indeed when he was involved in the development of the Ottawa Charter. Potvin, is from the province of Québec, the French speaking part of Canada, which is also an area culturally very close to Europe, especially in terms of the development of Public Health in the 1980's. Finally, Kickbusch has spent most of her training and career years in Western Europe having come momentarily to the US to take on an academic appointment at Yale between 1998 and 2004. Conversely our European colleagues have all made extensive stays in the US. Balbo spent one year in Berkeley as one of the first female Fulbright scholars from Italy and was later a visiting professor at the University of California, Santa Cruz. Abel did his PhD at University of Illinois after a first degree in Sport Science in the Federal Republic of Germany. Pelikan completed a postdoctoral fellowship at Columbia University, New York. Although general conversations in our group were obviously carried out in English, the only language everyone understands and speaks, side conversations were also held in German and in French. More interestingly for the book, between the six of us we were able to access in the text, the major authors in contemporary sociology and this is reflected in the rich diversity of sources that are proposed in the reference sections at the end of each chapters. Key authors from France, Germany, UK and the US are abundantly quoted and referred to, which is somewhat unusual in public health and health promotion texts.

We are all well aware that the idiosyncratic composition of our group is paramount in the final product of the book. Other people would have tackled the task differently and would have come up with another book. It is interesting to note here that none of the people first approached by McQueen and Kickbusch declined their invitation. There is no second choice among our group. Of course there should have been an implicit rationale for selecting the people they did. However, since criteria were reconstructed after the fact, their validity is greatly questionable. Nonetheless, it seems that the most important one was the desire to work with and the anticipated pleasure to share texts and ideas with everybody.

4. Converging Trajectories

Each member of the group had a favourite theoretical tradition, and his or her preferred thinkers. Our early meetings focused upon these authors' theories and their intellectual legacy. Subsequently, while linkages and connections were developed and the scenario of health (and health promotion)—that many of these authors had obviously not considered—came to the fore, some of these contributions were dropped, while others became crucial parts of our common background. This progressive process was slow, and somewhat difficult to cultivate at the early stages. Lively discussions, challenging lines of reasoning and hypotheses, were frequent characteristics of our dialogue. One's intellectual practices, or we might even say one's intellectual identity, were occasionally under friendly attack.

The process also brought about a fruitful convergence among participants, active in, and informed about, health promotion issues and practices in different contexts and institutions. Past developments and recent contributions in the field were either criticized or shared and taken into consideration with insightful analyses. There were at certain moments, privileged bilateral exchanges; during the meetings a plural confrontation and dialogue always developed. Our sense of membership also developed through several opportunities in which we were invited as a group and had to act as such in front of different external audiences. In 2002 and 2003, we did consult twice with the Swiss Foundation for Health Promotion in Bern. In

Montreal, in 2003, we had a working session on the orientation and evaluation of Fondation Lucie et André Chagnon's community mobilisation program. Finally, at the XVIIth IUHPE (International Union for Health Promotion and Education) meeting held in Melbourne in 2004, four of us presented our work in a session on theory in health promotion. After the fact, we recognise these meetings as important landmarks in the development of our common view of health promotion. We have come to be recognized as a group, i.e. as sharing common theoretical frames, perspectives, and languages: a common project.

At the end of the day our enterprise turned out to be a success story, in that a shared platform and understanding of the key role health promotion is playing in contemporary health agendas, as well as in the shaping of western societies, has emerged. It is also interesting to note that during the years of preparation for the final versions of our contributions we all obviously pursued parallel activities (academic engagements, conferences, writing on different topics, etc.) while keeping the "theory book" project in mind. This contributed to a process of nurturing insights and ideas for the project itself.

The stage of the actual writing was somewhat painful, in that several subsequent versions were thoroughly analyzed by each member of the group with the aim of improving convergence, clarity, and innovation. Questions and criticisms were sharp. There was a lot of homework between meetings: much re-writing, re-arranging, and reconsidering what each of us had initially taken to be a satisfactory product. It is not surprising then that at the end of our work, the various pieces that compose our book resonates with each other, and this despite the fact that a single author wrote each and that there was no attempt at unifying different personal styles of writing.

The result of all these meetings and conversations is, as you will notice, a coherent conception of health promotion and its role in, and relationship with, contemporary societies. As an echo to our modern world this cohesion was never deliberately organised from a master plan. It has grown through a process in which each of us gave and took. This would not have happened if people had just been assigned the task of writing a chapter on a particular subject.

One final word about the context of our work: although we had our first meeting in January 2002, after September 11, the society in which the health promotion we are talking about in this book is continually evolving in many ways that are relevant to the present discourse. New risks often framed as health threats have suddenly appeared, mobilising public health institutions in the process and reinforcing the health protection functions often at the expense of others. A radical change to pre-September 11 is the awareness that these new risks are not the unforeseen consequences of our technical interventions on nature as in Beck's description of the risk society. Most of these new risks result from deliberate actions that reorient medical and heath scientific knowledge into instruments of terror (Wright, 2004). These are profound changes in our societies' collective experience of health and they make even more critical our modest attempt at initiating a dialogue between health and those sciences that seek to reflect on society.

5. Concluding Comments

The writing of this chapter comes at this project's end. Our individual contributions to the fields of health promotion, social sciences and our personal trajectories can easily be retrieved from the WEB and through various databases in public health and sociology, but this is not what this book is about. What is really important is who we are as a group and how we managed to develop this book, addressing health issues as central questions through which we are able to further our understanding of society.

Throughout the process described above each of us was able to explore areas and ideas that were unknown or at least only very loosely formulated when we signed on for this journey. It has been a new way of generating knowledge and introducing a more dynamic way to learn: in fact, it has, and is a win-win experience.

References

Frohlich, K. L., Corin, E., & Potvin, L. (2001). A theoretical proposal for the relationship between context and disease. *Sociology of Health and Illness, 23,* 776–797.

Glanz, K., Rimer, B. K., & Lewis, F. M. (Eds.). (2002). *Health behavior and health education: Theory, research and practice* (3rd ed.). San Francisco, CA: Jossey-Bass.

Kickbusch, I. (1986). Life-styles and health. *Social Science & Medicine, 22,* 117–124.

McLeroy, K. R., Steckler, A. B., Simons-Morton, B. G., & Goodman, R. M. (1993). Social science theory in health promotion. *Health Education Research: Theory and Practice, 8,* 305–312.

Williams, G. H. (2003). The determinants of health: Structure, context and agency. *Sociology of Health & Illness, 25,* 131–154.

Wright, R. (2004). *A short history of progress.* Toronto: Anansi.

3
Modernity, Public Health, and Health Promotion
A Reflexive Discourse

LOUISE POTVIN AND DAVID V. MCQUEEN[1]

1. Introduction

Reflecting on the nature of evidence produced with regards to health promotion, one of us (McQueen, 2001) recently argued that health promotion could not yet claim the status of a scientific discipline. One symptom for this, McQueen noted, was the absence of a largely agreed upon corpus of theoretical concepts and propositions that would rally those who are engaged in the discourse or in the practice of health promotion. In established science, such a corpus makes the content of introductory textbooks and as a consequence of the large consensus about the objects and methods that constitute a discipline, the table of contents of most contemporaneous introductory textbooks are very similar. Such consensus and the accompanying uniform content are still lacking in health promotion, and it is certainly not our intention that this book should become one. Quite the contrary, our aim with this book is to offer for discussion a theoretical perspective for health promotion. Such a theoretical perspective, we argue, is necessary to support exploring the role of health promotion in contemporary society and to inform our response to the challenges facing the development of the health promotion knowledge base and practice. These are necessary conditions if health promotion is to evolve into a profession (see Pelikan, Chapter 6).

Over the roughly quarter century of its young history, the issue of a theoretical basis for health promotion has come up regularly. Interestingly, however, very few among those contributions seemed to be in associated with the theoretical discussions that were taking place in the preparation of the 1986 meeting in which the Ottawa Charter was adopted. As the codification of a field and the institutionalization of a given discourse, the Ottawa Charter,[2] with its five strategies for action does not make strong references to its own theoretical underpinnings. In addition

---

[1] The findings and conclusions in the report are those of the author(s) and do not necessarily reflect the views of the Centers for Disease Control and Prevention.

[2] The term Charter is itself a strong statement about the official and institutional nature of the propositions contained in the Ottawa Charter. It is a short document aiming at a broad and diverse audience with a clear goal of orienting action.

to the Charter itself that was a product of the conference, the group of scholars and public health officials involved in this endeavour also produced two major documents. The first one often referred to as the "Concepts and Principles" document is relatively unknown and was mostly circulated by the working group members.[3] The second paper was an article published in 1986 in *Social Science Medicine* (Kickbusch, 1986). Although it was available for a potentially larger diffusion than the "Principle" document, it is rarely cited in relation to the Ottawa Charter. Meanwhile, in the past two decades the Charter has acquired a life of its own.

Going back to these two documents twenty years later, one is struck by the fact that together they provide a solid foundation for the development of a knowledge base and a professional practice for health promotion with a strong emphasise on the paramount role of the social organisation of life in the making of health for both societies and individuals. "A new perspective is needed on lifestyles, one which places them firmly in the context of broad social trends and defines them as inherently social in origin and in growth" (Kickbusch, 1986, p. 124). The framework for health promotion actions according to the "Principle" document is formed by the health inequalities that follow from social inequities. The knowledge base for those actions should be multidisciplinary, making a large place for theories that help to understand the functioning of society and how change occurs and can be oriented. Finally both these documents situate health promotion in the continuity and a development of public health and conceived it as the public health answer to the challenges posed by our changing society.

In a sense, this book takes up where those two documents ended twenty years ago. Collectively reflecting upon the role and meaning of health and health promotion in our contemporary society, our group proposes that health promotion has been implicitly elaborating a discourse and a practice for public health in modernity. This book is about providing categories in which one can reflect that discourse and practice. Before doing so however, we felt a need to map out what, as a group, we agree to consider as the starting point of our search. This chapter presents what we believe the core of the field that we call health promotion looks like.

2. Health Promotion: Neither a Profession Nor a Discipline

For many in health promotion, the Ottawa Charter provides the founding characterization of the field of health promotion.[4] The World Health Organization's

---

[3] This document was produced and printed as a "taxi" document, meaning it was designed to be given out when someone, metaphorically traveling with one in a taxicab, would ask what health promotion was all about. Many copies were distributed, but few original copies of this printed document probably remain extant. We reproduce this document as an appendix of this book so it can be widely available and placed in historical context. The enormous progress of sociology regarding the structure/agency issue and the radical transformations of our society following the fall of communism and the acceleration of globalization could not be foreseen by the documents' authors.

[4] No doubt the Charter has gained wide currency since its formulation. It was the consensual product of a limited group of people, meeting in Ottawa, interested in health promotion. No

based Charter essentially offers an orientation for public health action along five strategies.[5] For us, the Ottawa Charter, together with its accompanying documents, represents the first attempt to codify an approach to public health practice that has been developing since the 1970's[6] in response to the profound transformations that Western societies were experiencing. In other words, we understand health promotion as a strategy for public health that reflects modernity. That strategy was developed and formally adopted in the beginning of the 1980's. Although initially it was rapidly infiltrating many government agencies and public health organisations throughout the world, this institutionalisation process has slowed down in many jurisdictions. It is not that the idea, principles, and strategies of health promotion are no longer relevant or implemented in public health practices, but rather that the term "health promotion" itself, as the denomination of a sector of activities such as government branches or agencies, seems to have become outdated in countries like Canada and the UK. So paradoxically, although a lot of the growth in health promotion has taken place in institutions, it has not yet developed into institutional recognition, neither as a science nor as a profession.

Of course some people would strongly disagree with this point of view, citing the establishment of departments of health promotion, offices of health promotion, and other examples of "names on the door." However this phenomenon appears to be rather short lived and in more recent years there have been concerns among many practitioners of health promotion that the budding institutionalization of the field is rapidly disappearing. To a large extent health promotion is being seen as a generalizing principle of approach that is literally a good thing when it operates across all the dimensions of a public health institution.

Although a fair number of people who claim the identity of health promoters would also legitimately declare that of scientists, in light of their fundamental training in a discipline-based academic degree, most would agree that health promotion itself is not a scientific discipline. There are still too many debates on what is health promotion about (topics and themes of interest), about the epistemological posture appropriate for developing the knowledge base of health promotion and about the methodological apparatus to be deployed to produce that knowledge. In addition, health promotion is still lacking the institutional tools that would make it recognized as a science. For example, there exist only a few health promotion

---

document, no matter how carefully constructed, can claim to be all inclusive and capture every interest in an emerging field. Nonetheless, it represents the only document that is a product of several discussions, workgroups and deliberations held by groups of concerned individuals representing multiple disciplines and perspectives. In that sense it was created in the spirit of health promotion.

[5] For those readers less familiar with the Ottawa Charter, those strategies are: 1) developing personal skills, 2) fostering supportive environment, 3) strengthening communities, 4) reorienting health systems, and 5) developing healthy public policy.

[6] Indeed, the Canadian policy document entitled "Perspective on the Health of Canadian" that was presented by the then Canadian Minister of Health Marc Lalonde, is often cites as one of the important building block & for health promotion, together with the WHO Alma Ata Declaration of 1978 that established the global goal of "Health for All in the Year 2000".

departments in universities, therefore diplomas in health promotion, whenever they exist, are usually sub-specialties of other degrees, most often in public health but also in nursing or in psychology. Despite this lack of institutional credit, there are some indications that health promotion knowledge is gaining recognition. The number of scientific journals dedicated to health promotion continues to grow, as well as the number of research centres and academic units that use health promotion in their title. Those centres and units often include scientists from various university departments together with researchers appointed by organisations from the health system, reflecting the fact that the scientists engaged in the production of health promotion knowledge do so from a multi-disciplinary perspective, mainly found in the health or in social sciences. As an interdisciplinary field, health promotion has yet to reconcile the theoretical and methodological perspectives that were only rarely brought together to look at the same reality.[7]

In addition, we believe that health promotion is not strictly a profession per say, and several reasons support this assertion. Firstly, a lot of what we consider health promotion practice occurs totally outside of the codified professional world. In countries like Switzerland, Canada and Australia, private and public foundations fund cutting edge health promotion projects designed and implemented by community organisations that are composed of 'lay people' with little professional training. Interestingly, some of these projects have lead to real social innovations when properly nurtured by caring funding and/or research institutions. Secondly, there are few organisations dedicated to the professional advancement of health promotion. Those who engage in health promotion practice regroup either in special sections of broader professional associations such as in the Public Health Education and Health Promotion Section of the American Public Health Association (see www.jhsph.edu/hao/phehp), in associations where they are paired up with other professionals occupying overlapping fields, such as in the International Union for Health Promotion and Education (see www.iuhpe.org), or on a project basis in a loose network such as the Réseau francophone des intervenants en promotion de la santé (see www.refips.org). Thirdly, there is very little consensus on what would constitute a health promotion practice and this is evidenced by the persisting debate about whether health education is part of health promotion. It is also illustrated in the failure to establish licensure and professional practice guidelines for the field. In short, almost anyone, trained in any discipline, who wishes to take on the moniker of "health promoter" may do so without fear of censure or disapproval by a standardized professional body.

We think that it is important at this point in the evolution of our field to reflect on the meaning and consequences of this lack of a distinctive institutional structure for health promotion, and whether it is important to develop one such structure. The absence of a distinctive structure certainly makes health promotion more

---

[7] One could argue that sociology of medicine had brought together disciplines from these two fields. This is only partly true because they were not looking at the same object. In fact, in sociology of medicine the latter forms the object of enquiry of the former. This is a debate that goes well back to the 1960's debate on sociology "of" versus "in" medicine.

vulnerable to decisions made by others, particularly with regard to the power to dictate programmatic directions. The difficulty to secure funding for research and programs in health promotion is certainly a consequence of this vulnerability. The main response that health promotion has formulated to this threat has resulted in attempts to justify its existence by documenting the effects on some outcomes valued by policy makers and public health decision makers, from where most of its budget comes.

The absence of a distinctive institution also has certain advantages. The most obvious one is that those who engage in health promotion activities enjoy a greater freedom to innovate and experiment on new ways of addressing the problems raised by living in our society. In a little more than two decades, health promotion has been a formidable laboratory for designing and experimenting with new and innovative ways to address emerging and challenging public health issues. Some such programs that have been identified as inventive approaches such as healthy cities, healthy schools, health promoting hospitals have spread throughout the globe and have greatly contributed to the dissemination of the idea that health is produced and maintained in every day life. Moreover, these programs have also contributed to a profound reorientation of practice in the institution of public health. Instersectoral action, healthy public policy, population health assessment, public participation and the new governance, all those practices that are now integrated to various degrees into the institutional discourse of public health (see for example: The Swedish Health Policy Statement: Health on Equal Terms; The Québec National Public Health Program; The Pan Canadian Healthy Living Initiative), were initially introduced through health promotion programs and projects.

So if it is not a discipline, nor a profession, nor an institution what is health promotion? At the very least, health promotion is a structured discourse and a set of practices or what has been termed a "field of action" (McQueen, 2001). The increasingly numerous journals in which health promoters articulate a discourse and disseminate their ideas, together with the burgeoning number of conferences where health promotion issues are discussed and debated, is a sign that an original discourse is being elaborated upon and incorporated into other contemporary public discussions. Two features stand out from this dialogue: the emergence of a distinctive perspective on health; and a critical orientation towards action. It is notable that it took two outsiders from the field to identify these two gems in the crown of health promotion. Indeed, the epidemiologist Lester Breslow (1999) articulated the health promotion concept that health is a resource for everyday life and fuelled what he termed "the third revolution of public health". At about the same time, the sociologist-epidemiologist Len Syme, in a report commissioned by the Institute of Medicine, recommended that in order to improve population health, public health should modify its practice in a direction that has been widely advocated by health promotion practitioners (Smedley & Syme, 2000).

So as a discourse and a practice, although neither a scientific discipline nor a profession, it seems that health promotion has much to offer to the very well established field of public health. To take Breslow's words, it is nothing less than a "third revolution" and it is our contention that the renewal of public health that health promotion is leading is much more profound than being only related to a conception of health.

3. The Third Revolution of Public Health

Several authors have used the revolution metaphor to describe the evolution of public health since the middle of the 19th Century (Susser & Susser, 1996; Terris, 1983), indicating that changes occurs in the field of public health through dramatic reorientations. To deserve the label of revolutionary such changes must affect the three fundamental dimensions that characterize systems of actions, such as public health: the direction or the finality of the system; its knowledge-base; and its practice (Potvin and Chabot, 2002). The finality establishes the target of the actions together with the set of objectives and goals that the system aims to achieve. The knowledge-base is both the substantive knowledge and the conditions that make possible the production of this knowledge about what constitutes the target of actions. The practice dimension encompasses the approaches developed to designing, implementing, and evaluating the actions that are necessary to attain the goals.

Terris (1983) identified two such revolutionary changes: the infectious disease and the chronic disease revolutions, and each of them can be described in terms of a dramatic change in finality, knowledge base and practice of public health. In addition to the traditional responsibility of the State to protect the health of its citizens, the infectious disease revolution pursued the goals of controlling and eliminating the threat posed by the great epidemics that had until then decimated human populations and prevented a steady and stable demographic growth. The knowledge base that fuelled this revolution was provided by the emerging and fast growing life sciences such as bacteriology, physiology and social statistics. While each of these disciplines was necessary to understand and address all aspects of transmissible diseases, one of the great achievements of the first public health revolution was to be able to integrate all these widely different knowledge into a coherent and comprehensive model of health and disease. In terms of practice, this first revolution was no less dramatic. Public health was no longer left to the initiatives of charity organizations or as an ad hoc answer to an emergency situation; it became integrated within the bureaucratic regulatory system that the nascent Nation-State was elaborating (Fassin, 1996; Porter, 1999). The complexity of the task at hand and the enormity of the means that were necessary for its completion required the mobilization of the resources of entire nations. This integration of the burgeoning scientific knowledge of life sciences with the population management capacity of the Nation-State provided to public health a jump start for the establishment of a practice founded on the authority of expert knowledge in the service of the common good.

Once transmissible diseases were mainly under control, chronic diseases became the leading causes of death, forcing a second revolution for public health. The fact that the majority of children lived to adulthood, and that women were surviving childbirth were all incentives for embarking upon a new goal for public health, that of increasing human longevity through the prevention of chronic diseases. The knowledge base of public health grew with the integration of the rapidly expanding clinical sciences. The fight to cure chronic diseases has been stimulated by, and has stimulated in return, the development of experimental medicine and a plethora of bio-medical science sub specialties. The practice of public health has been transformed by a deep professionalisation movement. It became integrated in the established medical professions, such as physicians and nurses and a range of other emerging ones such as health educators, rehabilitation specialists, nutritionists and so on.

In a recent paper, Lester Breslow (1999) argued that the emergence of health promotion and the development of the Ottawa Charter for health promotion are signs that the field of public health is undergoing a third revolution. For Breslow, the fact that in many countries human longevity is reaching its upper limit and that individuals expect to live a long life relatively disease free, is demonstrating a shift in the public health agenda so that "some energy can now be devoted to advancing health in the sense of maximizing it as a resource for living," (Breslow, 1999, p. 1031). So health is no longer conceived simply as a "biological" feature of the human life, but a product that one should possess for as many years as feasible. Produced in everyday life, health encompasses all aspects of life. Defining health with such a comprehensive perspective requires an expansion of the current knowledge base, which is also characteristic of the third revolution (Potvin, Gendron, Bilodeau & Chabot, 2005).

If health is produced in everyday life then intervening on health requires knowledge about how individuals in society make decisions and act in a way that affects their health in their everyday life. Conversely it also necessitates an understanding of how societies change through the actions of, and inter relations among, those who constitute society. The production of health in everyday life also means that experts should come to a new understanding of their role. Their expertise has to become relevant in the management of everyday life. These new requirements regarding experts' role are reflected in the realignment of the knowledge base for public health. First, in terms of scientific disciplines, there is a greater integration of knowledge from a wider range of the social sciences, some even questioning the epistemological foundations of epidemiology (Potvin et al., 2005). Second, lay knowledge is also increasingly valued as a legitimate source of knowledge that should complement scientific knowledge in the construction of evidence to support or evaluate action (McQueen, 2001).

Finally, in line with the integration of lay knowledge, the third revolution of public health is associated with a change in practice that is characterized by: 1) a strong reliance on citizens input and participation in decision making regarding health and public health interventions, 2) an integrated approach that both targets a variety of interrelated risk factors and the social conditions with which they are associated, and deployed activities in a multiplicity of settings.

These changes in the definition of health, along with changes in the knowledge base that is the foundation for interventions, and in the practice of public health have been heralded in the health promotion discourse since its inception. In all these, health promotion has been avant garde and leading the way for public health. The dialogue between health promotion and public health is well established in the field, and there are many examples of its fruitfulness. In its National Public Health Program for 2003–2012 for example, the government of Quebec identifies health promotion as one of four core function of public health, at the same level as prevention, protection and surveillance (Health and Social Services Québec, 2003). In its Pan Canadian Healthy Living Initiative, Canada has clearly defined both the improvement of health and the reduction of health inequalities has two equally important overarching goals (Secretariat for the Intersectoral Healthy Living Network, 2005). In addition, the strategies called for "integration" and for "partnership and shared responsibilities" as guiding principles for the Initiative. Finally, the "Health on Equal Terms" Swedish health policy identifies as the five priorities determinants of health that lie in the social realm (Swedish National Committee for Public Health, 2000).

We strongly believe that public health constitutes an obvious institutional niche for health promotion. There is increasing evidence that at least in its spirit, the health promotion discourse and practice have permeated deeply into the discourse and practice of public health. As a consequence, it should be clear that those engaged in health promotion should have a good understanding of public health in order for health promotion continue to be a rich field for innovation and experimentation for public health. Conversely, health promoters should also have a good grasp of what is distinctive about health promotion.

4. Conclusion

One of the main thesis underlying this book is that in its short history, health promotion has not paid enough attention to theories of the social science. The health promotion discourse has not been able to adapt and develop the proper tools to reflect upon the theoretical bases of what constitute its distinctive added value to public health. The third revolution of public health identifies that health is recognized as a social phenomenon as well as a biological and psychological one. Public health, therefore, should engage in a sustained dialog with social science and consider not only borrowing its methods and instruments, but also some of its theoretical understanding of the world, and how it shapes human action. One of the important roles for health promotion is to be the interface and to provide a space for this dialogue to happen between public health and the social sciences.

In the field of public health, social epidemiology also claims to set up bridges between social sciences and public health. Several influential social epidemiologists hold graduate degrees in sociology and health economists were instrumental in the elaboration of the population health discourse that many falsely attribute to social epidemiology. Our position is that there is a lot of room for diverse bridges between the social sciences and public health. We do not claim this land for the exclusive use of health promotion; neither do we think that it uniquely belongs to population health or to social epidemiology. Our stand is that the same way that social epidemiology is ideally equipped to explore the role of the social determinants in the making of the population's health, health promotion is uniquely positioned to bring to public health a social science informed understanding of its practice, of its role as a social institution and on the significance of health in our contemporary society.

References

Breslow, L. (1999). From disease prevention to health promotion. *JAMA, 281,* 1030–1033.

Fassin, D. (1996). *L'espace politique de la santé*. Paris: Presses universitaires de France. Health and Social Services Québec. (2003). *Le programme national de santé publique du Québec, 2003–2012*. Downloaded March 27, 2006 from www.rrsss12.gouv.qc.ca/documents/Programme_nationale_sante_pub.pdf

Kickbusch, I. (1986). Life-styles and health. *Social Science & Medicine, 22,* 117–124.

McQueen, D. V. (2001). Strengthening the evidence base for health promotion. *Health Promotion International, 16,* 262–268.

Porter, D. (1999). *Health, civilization and the state*. London, UK: Routledge.

Potvin, L., & Chabot, P. (2002). Splendour and misery of epidemiology for evaluation of health promotion. *Revista Brasileira de Epidemiologia, 5*(Suppl. 1), 91–103.

Potvin, L., Gendron, S., Bilodeau, A., et al. (2005). Integrating social science theory into public health practice. *American Journal of Public Health, 95,* 591–595.

Secretariat for the Intersectoral Healthy Living Network. (2005). *The integrated pan-Canadian healthy living strategy*. Downloaded March 27, 2006 from www.phac-aspc.gc.ca/hl-vs-strat/pdf/hls_e.pdf

Smedley, B. D., & Syme, S. L. (2000). *Promoting health. Intervention strategies from social and behavioral research*. Washington, DC: Institutes of Medicine.

Susser, M., & Susser, E. (1996). Choosing a future for epidemiology: Eras and paradigms. *American Journal of Public Health, 86,* 674–677.

Swedish National Committee for Public Health. (2000). *Health on equal terms: National goals for public health*. Downloaded March 27, 2006 from www.sweden.gov.se/sb/d/574/a/17706

Terris, M. (1983). The complex tasks of the second epidemiologic revolution: The Robert Cruikshank Lecture. *Journal of Public Health Policy, 4,* 8–24.

4
Critical Issues in Theory for Health Promotion

DAVID V. MCQUEEN*

1. Why Have Theory in Health Promotion?

There are, of course, in the pursuit of science, all the classical reasons that stress the importance of theory. These will not be elaborated here because many do not apply to a field of work such as health promotion. Theory is probably most needed in order to help set the parameters for a scientific discipline, rather than a field of activity such as health promotion. Nonetheless theory serves a critical role in the conduct of most any activity and health promotion is no exception. Most critically, theory helps one avoid two types of error, one a narrow empiricism that concerns itself only with observation and the undirected collection of data and two an outlandish unanchored abstract thought that tries to address the entire range of understanding of the meaning of life. Health promotion practice is full of interventions, particularly at the community level, that are not anchored in any systematic theoretical approach. At the same time large conceptual ideas that are discussed in health promotion are equally found wanting an underlying theory. Finally theory anchors explanations in a field in the rich contextual efforts of many others who have thought long and hard about why social life is the way it is. A prime example is the discipline of sociology where a theoretical tradition has provided a rich source of explanation for phenomena ranging from socioeconomic status to globalization. To date there is no equivalent to this rich tradition in the field of health promotion. We have to create it.

At mid-century Robert Straus set out a critical distinction between sociology *of* medicine versus sociology *in* medicine (Straus, 1957). In an effort to categorize the activities of the budding field of medical sociology, he set out to distinguish between those sociologists who were steeped in the tradition of the sociological pursuit from those who applied their trade in the service of others. In my view one could draw a useful parallel to a theory *of* health promotion versus theory *in* health promotion. In particular this distinction could help in understanding the differing roles of the types of social sciences engaged in health promotion today. Part of this

---

* The findings and conclusions in the report are those of the author and do not necessarily reflect the views of the Centers for Disease Control and Prevention.

distinction relates to the distance one takes from the object of health promotion as a subject matter.

A theory of health promotion requires one to be removed a certain distance from the object of study and examine the very conceptual nature of health promotion; It is a more skeptical and critical point of view that is taken; It addresses fundamental questions about the concepts and principles of the field of health promotion. Theory in health promotion moves us much more to examine the application of theoretical perspectives in the day to day practice of the field of health promotion. Perhaps it is more reflexive and reveals more of the individual ideology of the practitioner. It is more sui generis. In the ideal world of discourse theories *of* health promotion could and would be derived by people outside of the field and be the subject of discussion by philosophers; whereas theories *in* health promotion would be generated by the practitioners of the art.

At the outset it should be made clear that this chapter, and indeed the approaches taken in most of this book, is more concerned with the notion of theory of health promotion than a theory or theories in health promotion. This point is salient because it is our belief that health promotion has been perceived as a field with little attention to theory because the emphasis has historically been on the application of psychologically based approaches in the practice of health promotion. This has resulted in a somewhat lopsided interest in the theories and theoretical approaches that apply to individual rather than group or collective behavior. A perusal of many introductory textbooks and readers finds a dominance of theories related to individual behavior change. Furthermore, these theoretical approaches are almost always initiated or applied in the service of a larger medicalized view of health promotion.

An example of the argument that public health and health promotion picked up the wrong end of the social science "stick", that is, the individual (micro) end rather than the social (macro) end, is found in a widely used model in health promotion called the Health Belief Model. The model was a heuristic device whose elaboration supported a plethora of research on the role of psychological factors in both the seeking of care and compliance with medical regimens. An earlier review of this activity was provided by Kirscht (1974) and a critical review by Norman (1986). The model was derived by social psychologists and rooted in the idea of "field theory" championed by Kurt Lewin and codified in work by Rosenstock (1974). In essence the model argued that participation in preventive health behavior can be predicted on the basis of an individual's perception of: (a) his susceptibility to a given disorder, (b) the seriousness of the disorder, (c) the benefits of taking action, (d) the barriers to action and (e) cues to taking action.

The emergence and subsequent wide application of the Health Belief Model in health education and promotion practice serves to illustrate further confusion between model and theory that characterizes much thinking in health promotion. "Model" and "theory" are often used synonymously in health promotion. The historic usage of the term "model" in mathematics and the physical sciences has generally been much more precise. That is, there is a model for a theory that consists of an alternative interpretation of the same purely formal axiomatic system of which the theory is an interpretation. If one takes the case of the Health Belief Model, it would be difficult to discover how a formalized theory was being articulated in the model. That is, the logical adequacy of the model is lacking. The discussion of models and their relationship to theory has been taken up by others in more detail (Achinstein, 1968, 2004; Bhaskar, 1997) and the relationship of scientific models to the social sciences by others (Henrickson and McKelvey, 2002).

The role of models in our discussion of theories in health promotion is important because generally speaking the level of theoretical discourse in the field is centered around "models" and "frameworks" rather than on direct theory. Furthermore the level of approach is generally at the micro level. The level of theoretical approach is an important consideration for health promotion theory as there is a significant disconnect between behavioral and social theories dependent on the level of the object. We possess a fairly well developed theoretical base of behavioral, psychological and socio-psychological behaviors as manifested at the individual level, but generally modeled. Similarly we possess a considerable body of theoretical literature stemming from sociology, anthropology, political science and economics that attempts to explain group, community, national and global phenomena. However, one could assert that there is little theoretical understanding of the relationship of these two levels, and, most critically, no theoretical perspective that explains both levels in a unified theory. Unfortunately, because of the ill-defined nature of health promotion both as a concept and a practice, the theoretical situation is very compromised, making the development of a theoretical perspective for health promotion very difficult.

Thinking about theory in terms of health promotion takes the reader towards the more macro approaches of social science. Because of this, chapters in this book address health promotion in terms of broader conceptual notions such as systems, modernity, globalization, and culture. In particular, this chapter considers health promotion theory in terms of several basic epistemological questions in the nature of inquiry in science and how these questions affect modern health promotion theory. This inquiry leads to explanations demanding theoretical approaches from the more macro social sciences as well as the natural sciences. From the social sciences the critical importance of the ideas of reflexivity and deconstruction has an impact on health promotion practice. Within the natural sciences, concurrent ideas of chaos and complexity severely challenge notions of how to carry out research and practice in health promotion and the implications for rethinking the theoretical base for the field and its everyday practice. Finally, the rise of the "evidence debate" (McQueen, 2002) impinges on the whole relationship between theory and practice in health promotion. The evidence debate helps to inform a theoretical way forward in a field marked by the need for proof of effectiveness and the generation of evidence-based models of best practice.

In considering the basis for health promotion theory, there is one overriding question: Is it possible to have a social theory of health promotion? This is a critical question because to a large extent health promotion is a "field of action" rather than a discipline. In addition health promotion may be seen as an ideology; raising the point that ideologies have beliefs as a basis, but rarely a theory. Particularly in the USA, health promotion practice has generally used a theoretical underpinning based largely on theories of behavioral change. As a result of this heritage much of present-day health promotion as a distinct entity in public health has rarely been concerned with theory.

2. The Everyday Practice of Health Promotion as a Challenge to Theory Building

Elsewhere it has been argued that health promotion is not a discipline in the sense that one generally refers to academic discipline areas, but rather a field of action or, in some instances, an ideological stance or "ethos" (McQueen, 1998). An academic discipline generally has a distinctive and consensual body of knowledge. There are numerous introductory textbooks to the discipline that are very similar in content; for example, basic chemistry or physics texts for high school or university. In these text books the content is rarely different; the emphasis is on presentation and learning of specific materials. An academic discipline has a general agreed upon conceptual framework—something akin to a loosely held theoretical position; it has agreed upon methods of inquiry into the key questions in the field; and it sets out a clear, generally logical pathway to discovery. This has consequences for theory building, theoretical explanations, and what is evidence for the field.

From a Kuhnian perspective, before a discipline develops it is in a pre-paradigmatic stage in which there is normally a long period of more or less directionless research into a loosely defined subject matter, there are various competing schools, with very different conceptions of what the basic problems of the not yet emerged discipline are and what criteria should be used to evaluate theories about that subject matter. Well-established disciplines rest comfortably in years, decades and often centuries of development of theory and the defining terms of practice. Thus they have had considerable time to define themselves as well as to define the basic elements of their field. Indeed, well-developed disciplines have defined and understood the primary elements of the field of study. It is argued that there is an accepted "received view" of the dimensions, content and boundaries of the field, a point well argued in Suppe's work on scientific theories (Suppe, 1977). Of course the notion of a "received view" is highly debated within philosophy of science and most would argue that at the height of the philosophy of science during the first half of the twentieth century there was wide agreement that scientific theories could be seen as "axiomatic calculi which are given a partial observational interpretation by means of correspondence rules." (Suppe, 1977, p. 3). This was the basis of the views of logical positivism underlying much of modern science at the end of the 19th and beginning of the 20th century. The implication is that we know what does and does not belong to a field of endeavor. Furthermore, the "received view" specifies clearly the methods to be used in the field and the criteria that must be realized to provide evidence that something belongs to the field.

Despite the power of explanation that is built into the notion of a "received view", it must be noted that the "received view" was only the acceptable paradigm for the collection of information that is in a scientific field. It was, in short, the best explanation for phenomena within the domain of the field at a point in time. In the latter half of the 20th century the writings of Hanson, Kuhn, Feyerabend and others (c.f. Suppe, 1977) challenged the received view and have in part led to the re-analysis and deconstruction of how science is conducted and how theories in science are manufactured. The critical point in this discussion with regard to theories of and in health promotion is that if one looks to the physical and so-called hard sciences for models for theory building, one must look beyond the time when the received view and logical positivism were dominant to the contemporary discussions of causality and complexity, (McQueen, 2000).

Depending on one's conception of health promotion it is either an ancient concern of medicine and public health or it is a recent phenomenon arising out of Western thought in the last quarter of the 20th Century. Both conceptions are probably valid, however as a distinctive conceptual presence in modern public health it is probably more recent and my position is that health promotion is essentially a modern ideology and has an underdeveloped "received view", let alone a sophisticated re-analysis and deconstruction of its underlying principles. Nonetheless, health promotion has become a major component of contemporary public health (McQueen, 2002 articles in Breslow book).

One challenge is to trace the major concepts and ideas that made health promotion the important component of public health that it is today. In the first instance this may appear to be an historical task, but theory plays a critical role. If one considers the history of any science, it generally starts with an insight into the theories that led to the development of the science. A discussion of the techniques and practices arising generally comes later. For example, in the history of the science of astronomy, one first sees the development of cosmological theories, that is, theories that explain why the universe exists, how it came into being, and why it is the way it is. These cosmologies are a kind of proto-science, they may even be characterized as ideology. Then follow the techniques of observation and exploration. Finally, one sees the applied use of the ideologies to define practical events, e.g. in the calendars, navigation, etc. Of course, the issue of which came first the descriptions of the heavens or the rationales for the heavens remains unknown. In reality these are probably not so separated. It is more likely that with the advent of writing and the development of the academic classes that the separation of theory and practice evolved. Thus, at some point in time, one arrives at a separation in the people who do theory from those who do practice. This separation seems to be historically common in the sciences and remains so today in many different forms, most notably the separation of engineering from science. The field of health promotion is no exception to this separation and it is this separation that makes the role of theory in the field so difficult to articulate; essentially health promotion is a field of practice that defined its role prior to defining its theory.

Normally a well defined discipline has, at a minimum, a hortatorical history and, with further development, a critical history. A sound history of health promotion as a field does not exist. Due to the relatively recent emergence of modern health promotion it has not developed a critical history within the field or any elaborate external history that would parallel the historical interest in medicine. Even the history of medicine has been more hagiography than history, which is just a simple historical description of who did what and when. For health promotion there has rarely been a critical look at the motivations of the practitioners, nor little appreciation for the political and social context in which the practice is pursued. The lack of a critical history makes the understanding and construction of a theory base for the field more problematic. One looks at history of a field to see how the various increments came into play that ultimately led to a clear definition of the field and an established paradigm leading to a theoretically based discipline.

Returning to the problem in discussing health promotion in terms of its history is the lingering problem of definition. To define health promotion is to state a theory of health promotion. Many have tried to define health promotion, but there is no agreed upon definition. It is not even clear who should agree on any definition. Efforts have been made to distinguish the concepts and principles of health promotion, and these efforts have been somewhat documented and at times addressed in a critical discussion (WHO (EURO), 1984). There have been efforts to describe health promotion in terms of the new public health. (IUHPE, 2003). Furthermore there have been other efforts to build a consciousness about health leading to a health promotion that goes beyond the medical model. However this effort has been guided to a great extent by force of argument and persuasion as opposed to a link to any social science theory. It is safe to say that there is not a readily recognizable theoretical underpinning to the current concepts and principles of health promotion. What does it mean to use the name health promotion?

3. The Crisis of Identification: What Is in a Name?

In the broad area of public health, the concepts and principles of health promotion arose in the final three decades of the 20th century in part as a response to broad changes in public health. First, there was the recognition that the burden of diseases in the post industrial world had shifted predominantly to chronic diseases. Second, many asserted that the causes of these diseases were to be found principally in lifestyles and the social context, that the biomedical model of disease had severe limitations. Finally, there was increasing acceptance that health interventions had to address broad contextual factors such as empowerment, poverty, governance, health literacy and social capital. Health promotion was one response to these changes and remains so to this day, and because Universities bear the burden of reflecting the received intellectual currency of the times, health promotion departments appeared in those places where there was sensitivity to modern times. Of course it may be argued that traditional departmental structures in a University are not the best fit for an allegedly multidisciplinary field that constitutes health promotion. There are other alternatives such as Centers or units or other organizational, matrixed-type approaches. The issue remains pertinent when one considers theory, because where is the focal point for the theory of health promotion? In which organizational structure within academia would it be taught?

Are there any core disciplines that distinguish public health from health promotion? Based on a review of core subject areas in public health schools in the USA one can assert that the core disciplines of public health are epidemiology, biostatistics, behavioral and social sciences, environmental sciences, management and policy sciences, and biology. These are very inclusive of the broad range of practice of public health, but they also represent the disciplinary base of health promotion and hence its sources of theoretical underpinning. The special character of health promotion in terms of its concepts and principles is that it is multidisciplinary and cuts horizontally as well as vertically within these core disciplines.

Contemporary health promotion had its origins in the West. It was refined, developed, and institutionalized in Europe, North America and Australia, perhaps because these were the geopolitical areas to first come to grips intellectually with the consequences of modernity and its implications for health. Organizational, institutional and governmental responses to health promotion were manifested in the addition of health promotion to their agendas and in many cases to their name, but it remained for the academic world to recognize this field of action as a critical component of public health. In this context the establishment of Professorships in health promotion set a groundbreaking precedence. Such academic recognition was perhaps the leading edge of a budding discipline base; however, recent efforts to eliminate departments of health promotion in several universities argue for an erosion of this aspect, again signaling the lack of a disciplinary development, but rather the idea that health promotion is an area that cuts across disciplines. Therefore, there is a widespread view currently that health promotion has become such a fundamental component of public health that it does not belong to a single chair or a department, that it is ubiquitous and therefore its concepts and principles have been instilled throughout the education and practice of public health. This is laudable of course, but one must examine carefully why there is a name on a door. The name conveys the sense that this is the place where the fundamental values of an area of work or a discipline reside. For example, many in public health assert that epidemiology is the "science of public health," and indeed in the institutions, academic and governmental that carry out public health, one finds epidemiologists in every area of the institution. However, just because epidemiologists work throughout public health departments and epidemiological methods are widely applied by others, one still finds an epidemiology department with that name on the door. Organizationally there are departments with distinctive names because that is where the seat or the chair of the field is most and best represented, practiced and researched and where we look for both the fundamental substance of the practice as well as the future development of the field. The critical assertion here is that fields that have a name on the door have usually three distinctive components: one being a sound theoretical base, the second an historical development around a paradigm and a clear set of basic methodological criteria for how to carry out the practice of the field. In short, they have an agreed upon set of the critical questions in the field and an agreed upon set of methods as to how to go about answering those questions. These critical questions almost always arise from a theoretical base.

4. A Rough Interpretation of the History of Health Promotion: Theory and Practice

In the halls of public health academe some skepticism greeted health promotion in the early 70's, but this was soon replaced by a flurry of activity and transformation in the latter part of the 20th century in the world of public health. This transformation stemmed from many sources but notably there was the Lalonde report in Canada, Healthy People in the USA, the Ottawa Charter, the concern with a healthy public policy, the WHO (EURO) effort to develop the concepts and principles of health promotion, the Healthy Cities movement, (Cattford, 2004) to mention a few of the key historical steps to a more mature field of health promotion. Each of these steps in the development of health promotion aided in reducing the scepticism about health promotion and fostered the development of what was termed by some as the "new public health", a largely European movement in public health.

Whether or not there was health promotion before the 1970's is really a question of interpretation. Little doubt remains that in the generic sense public health since its inception has been concerned with promoting the public's health (McQueen, 1989). Nonetheless the term 'health promotion' largely dates from the 1970's and stems from several sources mentioned above and largely from the health field concept seen in the Lalonde Report that made health the focus of four factors: human biology, lifestyles, organization of medical care, and the environment.

The 1990's represented a watershed for health promotion. These years brought the challenge in which health promotion had to prove its utility to both the sceptics and those who have had their consciousness raised by the rhetoric of health promotion; this was the decade of the rise of the evidence question, or what I have termed elsewhere as the "evidence debate" (McQueen, 2002). The origins of this debate are found in a clinical medicine that sought to establish a dialogue on evidence-based medicine. Gradually this debate has been extended to health promotion and community-based public health interventions. The assumption is that this is an important and vital debate, that it is necessary to demonstrate what constitutes evidence and therefore proof that actions are effective. Although, the terms of the debate stem from clinical medicine rather than preventive medicine, the application of evidence criteria has taken evaluation down a path implying scientific rigor and justification. Evidence as a topic may be debatable, but arguably many health promoters desire to either justify their actions or demonstrate to others that their field of application is one with tangible benefits. Still, there are many, particularly in health promotion who believe that evidence, the very word, is inappropriate in evaluating much of public health practice.

What is most useful about the evidence debate is how it has served to illustrate the need for a theoretical basis for health promotion. The debate has made explicit the notion of contextualism. More than ever, health promoters are aware of the social and cultural context in which they carry out their work. This awareness applies at all levels of society. At the local level they are sensitized to local needs and public understandings of health. At the global level they recognize the incredible diversity of nations in terms of development, cultural beliefs, and governance.

Despite this accepted awareness of the great diversity in populations, some may still hold the belief that the evidence discussion is not affected by the contextual diversity. However, though many who are concerned are unaware of it, reflexivity has entered in to the evidence debate, in that those who have been engaged in the evidence debate now recognize that the cultural bias of the evidence discussion must be taken into consideration. Notions such as "evidence", "effectiveness", "investment", and "stakeholder", are rightly viewed as Western derived, European-American, and in many ways Western concepts. These concepts developed largely out of Western philosophical writings of the past two centuries and the epistemological underpinnings fostered by the development of logical positivism and were in essence a hall mark of modernism (Bhaskar, 1997). The idea of evidence emerging from experimental design is an historical product of this development, with the randomized controlled clinical trial (RCT) and the quasi-experimental approach largely creations of a Western literature. These approaches are widely accepted and almost universally applied in the physical and biological sciences, however, in the social and behavioral sciences their acceptance is less universal. Unfortunately many alternative approaches have not been so vigorously pursued. Nonetheless, there are rich theoretical underpinnings to the ideas in the evidence debate.

In turn, the view that there could be an evidence driven research base to health promotion introduces the question of a theoretical base and the linkage of health promotion to a broader theoretical context. That broader context was the rise and growth of health promotion as part of something bigger that was emerging in the domain of public health; a new kind of public health, and health promotion was at the core of this new public health; colleagues talked excitedly about 'paradigm shifts', a 'new social epidemiology' and the emergence of a new way to think about health and the public health.

5. Grand Theory Versus Many (Little) Theories

Brief mention should be made here about a theory of health promotion in contrast to many theories of health promotion. In this chapter it is assumed that *there is no obtainable unifying theory of health promotion*. While it is true that a particular approach to a particular health promotion problem might be inspired by a theory, or even be seen as a test of a theory, in almost all cases of this type the particular health promotion action would be only partially explained by any single theoretical position

6. What Is the Practice of Health Promotion and How Does Practice Relate to Theory?

Much of health promoting activity takes place in an organized context, principally the academic world or that of institutionalized government, even as health promotion practice may take place in a community, it follows from designs derived from, initiated by and supported by the academy and government. Just as the definition of health promotion helps define the theory of health promotion, the sponsoring institutions often delineate acceptable define the theory. Funding institutions are the primary settings for the development and initiation of the practice of health promotion and the source of the underlying methodological approaches. Even if the setting of application is a legislature, or a community, or a municipality, the development of the approach is most often developed, debated, the fundamental ground rules for the conduct of the practice stems from those in the institutional organization in which the field is practiced. The academy is not without implicit and explicit assumptions about how research and practice is conducted. With regard to theory, often there is the explicit expectation of a theoretical underpinning to any practice that is developed. That is the practice is explicitly linked to hypothesis testing, academic research, and often the writing of an academic paper and/or the preparation of a thesis or dissertation. An explicit characteristic of this type of academic pursuit is that it takes place within some academic discipline and the theoretical underpinning of that discipline. In any case, in even the most practical and atheoretical approach to any health promotion intervention, there are many implicit theoretical assumptions in the practice of health promotion. (E.g., even in the case of purely descriptive endeavours there are underlying assumptions about what to describe that is based in a theoretical perspective). Patterns of discovery do not arise from just observation, but rather from expectations about what is meaningful to observe. The choice of observation is ultimately dictated by theories implicit and explicit.

Location and context is meaningful; that is why the institutional setting for health promotion is so critical in terms of its theory. Elsewhere, I have written about what may be termed the "institution of research" (McQueen, 1990). This "institution" consists of a complicated mix of three components: (1) individual researchers: (2) research organizations; and (3) research funding bodies. Depending on the particular field of research, there is some agreement among the three components about what constitutes appropriate research. In the case of well established areas of research in public health, such as epidemiology, there is a relatively high degree of agreement about what constitutes appropriate subject matter and methodology within all three components. Put in a Kuhnian perspective, there is agreement on the puzzles to solve and the appropriate paradigms for research among researchers, research organizations and the funders of research. While there remains considerable debate and discussion about the nature of epidemiology and its appropriate role in public health, those who carry out research in epidemiology are supported by research organizations and funding bodies which share many ideas in common about research approaches. This situation is the direct result of a well established research paradigm and people being trained within that paradigm for decades. Underlying that paradigm is a consensual theory for practice.

Examples of institutional context are plentiful. If for example, the locus for health promotion is in a department of health education, then the theory base will be one of theories that focus on cognitive changes in individuals. Every institution, whether of government or academe, historically has assigned a place for health promotion. Thus if health promotion is seen as belonging to the noncommunicable or chronic diseases, then the health promotion programs will be heavily tied to the theoretical underpinnings of those who have been trained in chronic disease epidemiological approaches. If health promotion is seen as matrixed across an institution then the field will abandon a core theoretical focus.

7. Three Critical Conceptual Challenges Over the Past 30 Years, Each With Its Own Peculiar Implications for Theory Building and the Practice of Health Promotion

The first critical challenge is that of complexity. Complexity as a concept has two general forms, in the simplest form it alludes to the general difficulty to understand something and in a broader sense the degree of complication of something, for example a system or a structure, in terms of the number of components, intricacy, and connectedness of the structure. Many now recognize the complexity of social structures, social change, and the complex infrastructure that derives from the context of health promotion practice. There is a time-bound parallel of the currency of the idea of complexity with the development of health promotion. The idea of multivariate settings and situations is an idea that grew in part as a new way of thinking and in part in response to the ability of computers and statistics to handle multivariate problems. It is not that the world wasn't complex before the computer, but that the computer has allowed scientists to solve more complex problems. Health promotion picked up this profoundly different and emergent idea of complexity. Further, health promotion had to embrace complexity, rather than seek simplicity.

At the same time, there are forces that negate complexity. Simplicity is easier to argue than complexity because: a) cognitively, people want a single direct causal connection to an outcome (even if a group of people are complicit in the murder of a person, we want to know who killed the person); b) most causal models are conceived of as linear with discreet interconnecting causes (again, a product of earlier demands for simpler models that could be calculated by hand); c) traditionally science tends to be reductionistic in its relationship between theory and proof, stripping away complexity to understand the "true cause". Further the institutions and placement of health promotion has generally aligned with more traditional approaches to science and public health. Complexity is a real problem because it masks what many would like to see as the real or main reason why something happens. Further, there seems to be an innate need in people to understand precisely why something succeeds or fails. For example, in an aircraft crash, there is the search for the "black box" and when found the expectation that it will reveal the cause of the crash. There is always hope that it simply will be a bolt that was not tightened, or a circuit failed at a critical point. In reality such complex systems often fail because of multiple reasons, some knowable, some not. Even with a seemingly direct and simple causation, e.g. the bolt that was not tightened, one is left to address the problem of why it was not tightened.

However, complexity is an idea with many dimensions. It is not just the complexities of the subject matter itself that have arisen, but also the many notions of knowledge construction arising from the modern world. Many of these critical approaches actually question the nature of inquiry itself and not the substance of the field. For example, constructivism may be seen as an ideological recognition of complexity (McQueen, 2000). Partly this is because constructivism argues that one cannot separate agents and structures, that is, those who practice health promotion cannot be pulled back from the implicit theoretical constructions that they use. That is, actors socially construct (and deconstruct) the meaning of the ideas that they believe are primary in their field of action. This is not to present, at this point, constructivism as a principle of complexity, but rather to argue that constructivism is simply an exemplar of an idea that fits into the mix of what is emerging as the argument to consider complexity as a fundamental theoretical component of health promotion theory.

The idea of "contextualism" is a second critical challenge to theoretical considerations in health promotion. This idea may be anathema to theory building because it goes against the grain of the search for comparability and best practice. Obviously all human activity takes place in contexts; exploring the idea more deeply only adds layers to that observation and reveals how social actions are related to the context. The challenge is trying to grasp the meaning of contextualism when we want to relate it to a more profound theoretical understanding of human action. In particular we are challenged by the possibility that, try as one might, one cannot escape the inevitability of context and how it has forcefully shaped our understanding. Nonetheless, contextualism has revealed the limitations of logical positivism, the view that reason alone may lead to an understanding of society and ultimately the questioning of the nature of evidence itself. Thus the philosophy of science has moved relatively seamlessly from the ideas of Hempel, et al. (Suppe, 1997) to embrace those of Kuhn and followers. Further, contextualism has allowed cynicism, skepticism, relativism and deconstructionism to be seen as appropriate approaches to understanding the human condition. For health promotion, a field of action steeped in practice that occurs in a context, contextualism provides an approach to excuse the idea that there is any easy way to link practice to observation or observed effects that can be generalized. Indeed the principle effect of contextualism as an idea is not skepticism or hopeless complexity but its attack on the notion of generalizability. Further it argues that reality is directly in the context and not in a more abstract notion derived from theory. In turn this notion implies that it is the context itself in which consensus can be found. Many health promoters, practicing "in the field" have this notion almost as a mantra. If one argues that a health promotion program that works in Chicago couldn't possibly work in Jakarta because of contextualism, then it is ipso facto difficult to come up with a common theory of a health promotion program for large cities.

Finally, the notion of reflexivity is a critical challenge. In some ways it is an extension of contextualism except that the context lies primarily within the individual postulating a theory or and explanation. This is an elaboration of the concept as developed by Gouldner and others. Essentially the argument is that we frame or construct our theories based on our own biography. For example, if one develops a theory that is based on dynamism, accenting change over time, it is in response to a deep-seated inner need to understand why change occurs. But Gouldner makes another linkage on reflexive sociology that is relevant to this chapter: " ... those who supply the greatest resources for the institutional development of sociology are precisely those who most distort its quest for knowledge. And a Reflexive Sociology is aware that this is not the peculiarity of any one type of established social system, but is common to them all (Gouldner, p 498)." The parallel to the development of health promotion as a field and its institutions is clear. Health promotion, often leading by and defining itself as a field of action, often lacks apparent reflexivity. It is through a reflexive approach that the parameters of context and individual motivations are revealed, but also theoretical underpinnings are possibly revealed.

8. Additional Challenges of Gross Phenomena to Health Promotion Theories

Also, at the heart of health promotion theory and practice is the need to address some critical large scale phenomena of modernity. This is, in short, a broader scale dimension of the contextualism and complexity arguments. We recognize many large contexts that are critically important for health promotion, e.g.: Globalization; Urbanization; Degradation (environment); Pollution; Migration; Alienation; Immigration; Desertification; Population; and many others that may be on the reflective lists of others. It is not the intention to elaborate on these discrete and important topics.

One example of the problematic will suffice. Urbanization is a phenomenon that is dynamic and complex. It is, in general a recent phenomenon. Cities have existed for centuries and the city in history is well documented. However until the 20th century the planet was largely rural, prior to 1900 there were few urbanized areas greater than one million inhabitants; by the end of the 20th century there were many. When viewed from the perspective of history, this is an incredible and rapid change in the context of everyday life for almost every person living on the planet. What this phenomenon has done to cultural patterns based on the ideas of settlement, kinship, ethnicity, family, work, religion, communication, to name a few key sociocultural factors is a work in progress. That this enormous structural change is accompanied by global changes in health practices and outcomes is self-evident. Nonetheless the complexity of all the potential interactions at the micro to macro level presents challenges to health promotion practice and theory that need to be considered. Essentially can complex situations be addressed by simplistic strategies?

9. Complexity and Health Promotion Theory

Complexity has been considered in terms of its evolution as a component of late 20th Century thinking about science. Given that it has emerged a distinguishing feature of modern day thinking, the challenge is to consider whether the fundamental notions of complexity are related to and can be incorporated into health promotion theoretical thinking. Therefore this next section will consider some of the fundamental notions and place health promotion approaches in their context. Following that, the health promotion relationship to complexity in terms of modernity will be considered.

A fundamental notion of complexity is that the whole of anything is greater than the sum of the parts. This is certainly not a new notion, and is reflected in the idea that out of a multitude of simpler processes something unexpected may arise, often surprising, but in general different from anything that would have been predicted from a simple sum of the parts. While this notion appears as a good fit to health promotion theory and practice, it may also be argued that the "whole is the whole", that is simply that it is a whole entity and can only be understood in its wholeness. The implications for this notion are many, but most importantly imply that deconstruction is not a pathway to understanding of the whole.

The notion of complexity has many implications for health promotion theory as it relates to the notion of causality. To begin, causality itself has often been viewed or treated in a simplistic manner. To some extent this is because the initial parameters of causality were set by logical positivism to fit an emergent view of science that was based on direct linear cause and effect. Although the modern notion of causality can be traced to David Hume, this was not always the view. Nonetheless the Kantian tradition was more the approach that causality is just there, it is an *a priori* concept of understanding, that is pure concepts and pure intuitions shape our world, but tell us little about the things themselves. However the modern world transferred causality into a notion that demanded axiomatic structure, notions such as precedence of actors and a linear relationship to effect. Even more advanced notions of variables arranged in reciprocal and curvilinear causality remain essentially approaches based on logical positivism. Essentially, a contemporary health promotion eschews these recently derived notions and lead to the Kantian tradition.

The implication of rethinking causality in health promotion theory and aligning it to earlier as well as more recent thinking deriving from complexity is that causality is not totally knowable or perhaps even describable. This does not imply that causality cannot be understood, but that the understanding lies more with the interpreter of causality than with the events being described. Thus there is introduced a linkage between the notion of reflexivity, so prominent in late twentieth century sociological theory, and the understanding of causality in complex phenomena. For health promotion this is part of the foundation for tying together complexity, causality, and reflexivity as fundamental components of a health promotion theory.

The notion that the whole is the whole and that the whole is complex, challenges another fundamental procedure in the practice of modern science, namely the idea that a way or method to understanding of a phenomena (the whole in this case) is through reduction. The notion that the whole can be "reduced" to its components is fundamental to the idea of reductionism as developed by logical positivists. The assertion is that things are definable in terms of directly observable objects and that science is carried out by defining the terms in terms of increasingly more basic sciences. The assertion in this paper is that health promotion theory *can not be based on a notion that the whole can be reduced.*

A challenge for complexity and its role in an emergent theory of health promotion is that of systems theories. Certainly in its early formulations by Ludwig von Bertalanffy in the mid-twentieth century systems theories argued for a new analytical, methodological approach to dealing with the component elements of systems and in particular addressed the limitations of linear causality. Systems approaches introduced critical new concepts of interaction, transaction and understanding of relationships in multivariate systems. It certainly has been argued that general system theory is a general science of wholeness. Because of this the fit of a systems theory approach to health promotion has much to offer. However, the key epistemological question concerns the extent to which systems theories, however fashioned represent another form of reductionism and/or deconstructionism. The arguments for the case that systems approaches are the appropriate theoretical foundation are made in the chapter by Juergen Pelikan and will not be taken up further here.

Another feature that relates to complexity and health promotion is the distinction in science between that which is probabilistic and that which is deterministic. In the language of positivistic causality, most causal relationships, whatever their character, may be seen as deterministic, that is essentially that all causal relationships between variables are essentially knowable and could be determined if we had the appropriate measurements and had appropriately assessed all of the relationships. Just because determinism is difficult does not mean it is non existent. For example, the many-body problem in astrophysics may not currently be solvable, but essentially it could be solved. The idea that relations among variables are only knowable statistically is at the heart of most modern science as it is actually practiced. In a sense probability explanations are the best approximation of a complexity, given that we neither know nor have the skills or mathematical procedures to completely determine relationships in a complexity. In any case, at the present time, whether or not the universe and all things in it are knowable through either determinism or probability remains a philosophical debate. However, which approach a person believes to be most likely will influence the methodology sought to gain understanding.

A further notion related to complexity is related to the boundaries of a complexity, what is and is not in it and when. A concrete example of this is in the realm of interventions. When something is perceived as complex-a complexity- it has a certain wholeness. When a new parameter is introduced into that complexity, the whole changes. This is logical because something has been added to the whole. This added "part" may be seen as an "intervention". The epistemological question then becomes to what extent the whole has changed. Framed in this way, the reductionist, or approach to understanding what has happened is most appealing, primarily because one can then "examine" pre and post intervention how the whole or in turn its subcomponents have changed over time. Indeed, time and the dynamic of change appear to be the only relevant considerations.

Given that the notion of complexity is ancient, with origins at least back to the pre-Socratics, has modernity shaped the notion in any critically important way? To begin with, there is probably little doubt, given the vast outpouring of academic writing on the subject that quantitatively the discussion has greatly increased.

It is probably safe to assert that modernity has intensified the dialogue about complexity. However there are many possible tacks that have been taken, both implicit and explicit. For example, reflexivity, notably reflexive sociology recognized the role of the individual creative mind in the conceptualization of the social. In essence, as Gouldner ((1970) would argue, the social was not what was "out there", but what was "in here", that is in the sociologist's mind.

What exactly is the added value of the notion of complexity to health promotion and particularly to health promotion theory? That is a question with many answers and dimensions. Given that health promotion is conceptualized as a field of action, complexity provides the context for that action. Whether this is framed as "context" or "setting" merely makes the point that health promotion action does not take place on any part of a complexity, but always involves the whole. Secondly, given that interventions are made on a complexity, the theoretical notion of complexity makes the expectations of any action and potential outcomes more realistic. This is not an excuse for the general limitations and inabilities to easily see the fruits of an intervention, but a realization of how the complexity of the situation makes visibility of effect extraordinarily difficult to observe and/or measure. Thirdly, the notion of complexity provides important implications for evidence seeking efforts. The theory of complexity makes explicit that the "rules for evidence" lie in the reductionistic approach to science and that approach is inadequate to understanding and explanation in health promotion. Finally, complexity easily allows the introduction of a "values" perspective and base to action, thus reinforcing that component of health promotion that is ideological.

In sum, complexity as a concept appears to be an idea that should be critical in any theory of health promotion. While one could easily argue that the notion of complexity exists independently from modernity, the concept is both ancient and modern. More particularly the impact of discussions on complexity on late 20th Century science and philosophy has occurred at the same time as the rise of thinking in and about health promotion. In the history of ideas such seemingly parallel occurrences are seldom by chance.

Here it is important to state the overarching importance of complexity to health promotion theory. Health promotion is a field of action defined by its theory and complexity is the basis of that theory. However the primary implication of that theory is its relation to the practice of health promotion. This theory base moves the discussion of where theory should be placed. In this case, the theory drives the method (action) of health promotion, NOT the substance.

10. The Coterminous Dynamic Development of Health Promotion as Part of Larger Forces

To begin with, health promotion practice has been and remains difficult to define. It seems eclectic, encompassing a wide range of research types and approaches. Everything is relevant: policy research, evaluation research, survey research, action research, and social epidemiology. Many concerned with health promotion practice might disagree on the relative importance of the major areas for health promotion, but most would agree that there are critical issues with regard to the following areas: (1) theories and concepts in the field; (2) methodology and the whole issue of the "style" of research which is appropriate to practice; and (3) issues of application of findings, with an emphasis on translation of research and practice into something useful and oftentimes for the formation of policy.

Consider the critical issue of methodology in health promotion research. Even as the research methods used in health promotion have ranged from the qualitative to the quantitative, there is still unease as to what constitutes acceptable methods. Despite its apparent implausibility as a methodological approach suitable to health promotion, the RCT, or randomized clinical trial, remains for many who would term themselves health promoters, as an ideal to which health promotion research should aspire because it is seen by many as the method to use in evaluating drug trials, clinical interventions, etc. The lingering power of the RCT is witnessed in numerous debates and at meetings of health promotion. Despite forceful arguments to the contrary by leaders in health promotion evaluation, the RCT remains the bulwark for many public health practitioners that are either highly sympathetic to health promotion or would even classify themselves as health promoters. When control of the setting and population under study can be achieved for the time of the trial, and where there is a focus on a single intervention with an expected dichotomous outcome of success or failure, the RCT is indeed a powerful methodology, and there are those who argue fiercely that the RCT or a modified version thereof can at least be used for health promotion research (Rosen, O' Manor, Engelhard et al., 2006). Thus the post-modern separation implied by the rejection of a model like the RCT has not impacted on these researchers. Nevertheless, the strength of the RCT is directly related to rigidly meeting the restrictive assumptions of experimental design. When the severe restrictions of experimental design are not met, the utility, validity and power of the RCT diminish rapidly. The misapplication of the RCT in health promotion research is now legend.

In health promotion interventions, control and experimental populations are unlikely if not impossible. It is part of the very nature of health promotion interventions that they operate in everyday life situations, involving changing aspects of the intervention; outcomes are often decidedly different from expectations; unanticipated consequences of the intervention are common. Even if one rejects the strictest classical RCT model, the notions of experimental and control groups remains in studies and projects which use quasi-experimental designs, controls, and all the trappings of the RCT. Unfortunately, for many at the so-called hard end of the hard to soft science spectrum, a softer health promotion methodology seems implausible.

11. The Growth of Tradition and Ideology

Over the years different orientations towards public health have developed in the research community. Roughly speaking, a dichotomy exists between two traditions which could be termed "medical public health" and "social public health". These two traditions are not necessarily in conflict, but they often give rise to differing interpretations of the underlying mission of public health. Essentially, a public health steeped in the medical tradition tends to view epidemiology as the basic science of public health. It tends to view causation as linear and rely heavily on "evidence" gathered by a set of limited methodological approaches which use mainly experimental designs and a numerate tradition. Overall the stress is on the individual as the focus of public health programs with intent of influencing behavioural change. In contrast, a public health in the social tradition considers many disciplines to be relevant to research and places emphasis on the human sciences such as sociology, politics and economics. Causation is less relevant than patterns of change and complexity is expected.

Where does health promotion fit with regard to an orientation to public health research traditions? In my opinion, traditions are characterized as much by underlying ideology as in a strict adherence to the underlying disciplinary bases. Elsewhere I have argued for the emergence of an ethos of health promotion, which helps define the nature of the field. O'Neill, Rootman and Pederson (1994) talk about a "health promotion culture". I believe it exists, and that it is characterized by an ethos manifested through a debate primarily on methodology, but seldom on theory. Let me illustrate this assertion by going back to the watershed years starting in December, 1990 with the first national conference on health promotion research in Toronto. This conference was notable for several reasons. A number of papers and especially the keynote talks addressed fundamental problems in theory and methods for health promotion research. In short, issues presented at the meeting illustrated the emerging character of health promotion research. An international dialogue on health promotion research and practice took place, and that debate was centered upon the methodology of practice.

In part, as a result of this 10 year dialogue an 'ethos' emerged around health promotion research, which has research consequences: there is less emphasis on sophistication in quantitative analyses, and more on qualitative approaches. However the important point to note was that the debate generally focused on method. The argument was increasingly framed in post-modern terminology, for example one position is that sophistication in data analysis may have the effect of providing detail too elaborate or inscrutable for the general needs and use of public health workers and policy makers, introducing the paradox that some of the key notions such as dynamism, multi-disciplinary, complexity and context might demand rather innovative and complex data collection procedures and analyses, whether quantitative or qualitative. This ethos forced us to think again about theory and practice. Practice without theory can be seen as rudderless.

12. Theoretical Implications to Be Considered

In conclusion, the development of a theoretical perspective for health promotion presents many challenges that cannot be easily resolved. At the very least there are two fundamentally different bases for deriving health promotion theory. These arise initially by distinguishing between theory *in* versus theory *of* health promotion. However, it is not such a simple dichotomy, but rather one that derives its lack of clarity from the lack of definition of the field. We have rejected the idea that health promotion is a discipline and asserted that it is a "field of action". Fair enough, however that a field of action sometimes has a powerful ideological component and in other instances a powerful drive to be "scientific". This has consequences for what enters into the theory dialectic. When health promotion theory is concerned with conceptual ideas such as modernity, post-modernism, cultural capital, and other highly artificial constructions, one is taking the course of a theory of health promotion. It is concerned chiefly with explanation of the components that one is trying to change, rather than with the process of change. Furthermore, most of these components lie outside of the individual, they are a social product. On the other hand, when health promotion theory is concerned with change lying principally in the individual or a group of individuals, the road leads towards the theoretical explanation of experimental science. Thus the evidence debate becomes relevant for this type of theory. Unfortunately the concept of complexity operates at all levels and provides an underlying concept for health promotion theory, but it does not clarify the distinction between the types of theoretical perspectives. Further, if health promotion is seen as mainly ideological, driven by an ethos rather than a prototype theory, then it is unlikely that any unified theoretical base for health promotion will ever be reached.

References

Achinstein, P. (1968). *Concepts of Science: A Philosphical Analysis.* Baltimore: Johns Hopkins Press.

Achinstein, P. (2004). *The book of evidence.* Oxford: Oxford University Press.

Adrian, M., Layne, N., & Moreau, J. (1994). Can life expectancies be used to determine if health promotion works? *American Journal of Health Promotion, 8,* 449–461.

Allison, K., & Rootman, I. (1996). Scientific rigor and community participation in health promotion research: Are they compatible? *Health Promotion International, 11,* 333–340.

Appleyard, B. (1992). *Understanding the present: Science and the soul of modern man.* New York and London: Doubleday.

Beck, U., Giddens, A., & Lash, S. (1994). *Reflexive modernization: Politics, tradition and aesthetics in the modern social order.* Stanford, CA: Stanford University Press.

Bhaskar, R. (1997). *A realist theory of science* (2nd ed.). New York: Verso.

Bloor, D. (1991). *Knowledge and social imagery* (2nd ed.). Chicago: The University of Chicago Press.

Bunge, M. (1996). In praise of intolerance to charlatanism in academia. In P. R. Gross, N. Levitt, and M. W. Lewis (Eds.), *The flight from science and reason* (pp. 96–115). New York: New York Academy of Sciences.

Catford. (2004). Health promotion's record card: How principled are we 20 years on? *Health Promotion International, 19,* 1–6.

CDC, Internet site for the Community Guide: http://www.health.gov/communityguide.

Dean, K., & McQueen, D. V. (1996). Theory in health promotion. *Health Promotion International, 11*, 7–9.

Ehring, D. (1997). *Causation and persistence: A theory of causation.* New York: Oxford University Press.

EWG, European Working Group on Health Promotion Evaluation. (1998). *Health promotion evaluation: Recommendations to policymakers.* Pamphlet, WHO (EURO), Health Canada, Ottawa.

Gouldner, A. W. (1970). *The coming crisis of western sociology.* New York: Basic Books.

Gross, P. R., Levitt, N., & Lewis, M. W. (Eds.). (1997). *The flight from science and reason.* New York: New York Academy of Sciences (distributed by The John's Hopkins Press, Baltimore and London).

Henrickson, L., & McKelvy, B. (2002). Foundations of "new" social science: Institutional legitimacy from philosophy, complexity science, postmodernism, and agent-based modeling. *Proceedings of the National Academy of Sciences, 99*, 7280–7295.

IUHPE. (1999). The evidence of health promotion effectiveness: A report for the European Commission by the International Union for Health Promotion and Education, ECSC-EC-EAEC, Brussels–Luxembourg.

IUHPE. (2003). *The New Public Health: A collection of video conversation with people who shape our thinking about health and health care* (www.iuhpe.org).

Jammer, M. (1999). *Concepts of force* (2nd ed.). Mineola, New York: Dover.

Kirscht, J. (1974). Research related to the modification of health beliefs. *Health Education Monographs, 2*, 455–469.

Latour, B. (1987). *Science in action.* Cambridge, MA: Harvard University Press.

Latour, B. (1999). *Pandora's hope.* Cambridge, MA: Harvard University Press.

Latour, B. (2000). When things strike back: A possible contribution of "science studies" to the social sciences. *British Journal of Sociology, 51*, 107–123.

MacDonald, G., et al. (1996). Evidence for success in health promotion: Suggestions *for improvement.* In D. Leathar (Ed.), *Health education research: Theory and practice, 11*, 367–376.

McQueen, D. V. (1989a). Thoughts on the ideological origins of health promotion. *Health Promotion International, 4*, 339–342.

McQueen, D. V. (1989b). *Changing the public health,* Edited by Research Unit in Health and Behavioural Change (chaps. 1 and 2, pp. 1–28). Chichester: John Wiley & Sons.

McQueen, D. V. (1989c). *Schools of Public Health in den USA—Erfahrungen und Zukunftsperspektiven.* In B. Badura, T. Elkeles, B. Grieger, & W. Kammerer Zukunftsaufgabe Gesundheitsfoerderung, Landesverband der Betriebskrankenkassen in Berlin, Berlin, pp. 231–249.

McQueen, D. V. (1990). Comprehensive approaches to health research. In Evelyne de Leeuw, Chris Breemer ter Stege, & Gaspard A de Jong (Eds.), *Research for Healthy Cities, Proceedings of the International Conference on Research for Healthy Cities.* Supplement TSG 11/90, The Hague, pp. 52–58.

McQueen, D. V. (1991). The contribution of health promotion research to public health. *European Journal of Public Health, 1*, 22–28.

McQueen, D. V. (1994). *Health promotion in Canada: A European/British perspective with an emphasis on research.* In A. P. Pederson, M. O'Neill, & I. Rootman (Eds.), *Health promotion in Canada: Provincial, national and international perspectives* (pp. 335–347). Toronto: W.B. Saunders.

McQueen, D. V. (1996). The search for theory in health behaviour and health promotion. *Health Promotion International, 11*, 27–32.

McQueen, D. V. (1998). Theory or cosmology: The basis for health promotion theory. In W. E. Thurston (Ed.), *Doing health promotion research: The science of action* (chap. 3, pp. 29–40). Calgary, Alberta, Canada: University of Calgary Press.

McQueen, D. V. (2000). Perspectives on health promotion: theory, evidence, practice and the emergence of complexity. *Health Promotion International, 15*, 95–7.

McQueen, D. V. (2001a). Sociology in public health. In Lester Breslow, et al. (Eds.), *Encyclopedia of public health* (pp. 1132–1134). New York: MacMillan.

McQueen, D. V. (2001b). Strengthening the evidence base for health promotion. *Health Promotion International, 16*, 261–268.

McQueen, D. V. (2002a). The evidence debate. *Journal of Epidemiology and Community Health, 56*, 83–4.

McQueen, D. V. (2002b). Social and behavioral sciences. In Lester Breslow, et al. (Eds.), *Encyclopedia of public health* (pp. 1111–1116). New York: MacMillan.

McQueen, D. V., & Anderson, L. M. (2001). What counts as evidence: Issues and debates. In I. Rootman, M. Goodstadt, B. Hyndman, D. V. McQueen, L. Potvin, J. Springett, & E. Ziglio (Eds.), *Evaluation in Health Promotion: Principles and Perspectives* (pp. 63–81). Denmark: World Health Organization. (chap. 4, pp. 63–833). Reprinted in *Debates and dilemmas in promoting health: A reader* (2nd. ed.). In M. Sidell et al. (Ed.). Milton Keynes: Open University Press, 2002.

Norman, R. M. (1986). *The nature and correlates of health behavior.* Ottawa, Canada: Department of Health and Welfare.

Nutbeam, D. (1998). Evaluating health promotion—progress, problems, and solutions. *Health Promotion International, 13*, 27–44.

Poland, B. (1996). Knowledge development and evaluation in, of and for healthy community initiatives. Part I: guiding principles. *Health Promotion International, 11*, 237–247.

Rootman, I., Goodstadt, M., McQueen, D., et al. (Eds.). (2000). There is a shortage of evidence regarding the effectiveness of health promotion. *Evaluation in health promotion: Principles and perspectives* (chap. 24). Copenhagen: WHO (EURO).

Rosen, L., Manor, O., & Englehard, D. (2006). In defense of the RCT for health promotion research. *American Journal of Public Health, 96*, 18–24.

Rosenau, P. M. (1992). *Post-modernism and the social sciences.* Princeton, NJ: Princeton University Press.

Rosenstock, I. M. (1974). Historical origins of the Health Belief Model. *Health Education Monographs, 2*, 328–335.

Sackett, D., et al. (1996). Evidence-based medicine: What it is and what it isn't. *British Medical Journal, 150*, 1249–5.

SAJPM, Supplement to American Journal of Preventive Medicine. (2000). Introducing the Guide to Community Preventive Services: Methods, first recommendations and expert commentary. *American Journal of Preventive Medicine, 18*, 1.

Straus, R. (1957). The nature and status of medical sociology. *American Sociological Review, 22*, 200–204.

Suppe, F. (Ed.). (1977). *The structure of scientific theories* (2nd ed.). Urbana, IL: University of Illinois Press.

Tones, K. (1997). Beyond the randomized controlled trial: A case for A Judicial Review. *Health Education Research, 12*, 1–4.

Weiner, J. (1995). *The beak of the finch: A story of evolution in our time*. New York: Random House.

World Health Organization, European Regional Office. (1984). *Health promotion: A discussion document on the concepts and principles*. Copenhagen: WHO.

World Health Organization, European Regional Office. (1998). *Health promotion evaluation: Recommendations to policymakers*. World Health Assembly (1998) Resolution WHA 51.12 on Health Promotion. Agenda Item 20, 16 May 1998. Geneva: World Health Organization.

5
Cultural Capital in Health Promotion

Thomas Abel

1. Introduction: Health Promotion and the Unequal Production and Distribution of Health

Social inequality remains a key issue in health promotion to date. Empirical evidence on the role of material and non-material determinants of health and illness is mounting (Marmot & Wilkinson, 1999; Berkmann & Kawachi, 2000; Siegrist & Marmot, 2004). Under modern conditions of diversification and economisation in the health sectors findings from social epidemiology are essential to public health in general and health policy in particular. However, when examining social conditions relevant to the unequal distribution of health and illness, social epidemiology has traditionally focused upon either material conditions such as income, housing among others, or on social and psycho-social determinants such as education, social support, and psycho-social stress. Most often missing in public health research however, are cultural factors that link material and social resources, social structure and health. As health promotion focuses upon the development and maintenance of health in everyday life by the people themselves (rather than by medical experts), cultural factors become of central importance for theory development and practical interventions. For instance, health relevant behaviours are closely linked to broader value systems, behavioural norms, body perceptions among others, that may be typical for certain (sub-) cultures. They are adopted according to the environments in which people live, work and recreate and they are socially learned throughout the life course. However, from a sociological perspective the meaning of cultural factors is not limited to health relevant consumer choices for goods and services or explicit health and illness behaviours. Beyond such behavioural aspects, sociology has illustrated the crucial role that cultural factors play in the fundamental structuring processes of society (Max Weber, 1978; Durkheim, 1997; Giddens, 1991; Archer, 1996). Rooted in social science theory, more recent studies from medical sociology have linked health relevant values, norms and attitudes to social class; applying sociological theories to understand the emergence and consequences of health related lifestyles (e.g. Abel, 1991; Blaxter, 1990; Cockerham, Rütten & Abel, 1997; Frohlich, Corin & Potvin, 2001).

Health has long been understood if often only implicitly, as something given by nature or default, only to be restored or repaired, in the case of impairment or loss. However, one could also argue that, similar to wealth, health is something not merely "given by nature", but rather actively produced and maintained at all stages of life and in all dimensions in society. And in fact, all societies invest in health and healthy living conditions; and, different societies give varying value and priorities to the efforts to create conditions that support the active production of health. Applying the term "production of health" in health promotion attends to a current trend in modernity to promote health on the basis of deliberate and systematic planning. Today more than ever this implies the application of economic principles and rationales, such as the need for stringent target-oriented approaches, increasing value of health as a commodity in a rapidly expanding market, planned personal and social investments in health linked to deliberate return expectations.

Moreover, within modern societies, the production of and the investment in health are patterned along the stratification lines of gender, age, ethnical background and social class. Findings from social epidemiology have shown that the distribution of health is strongly—and often parallel to the distribution of wealth—linked to the underlying social structures of societies. However, public health knowledge into the underlying processes of the production of health remains weak.

As stated in Aaron Antonovsky's famous paradigm of Salutogenesis (Antonovsky, 1996), population and public health, from a health promotion perspective, can begin with positive health rather than illness or disease. Still, health promotion today appears to be torn between its new health centered paradigm on the one side and primarily illness or risk centered empirical data on the other. To date most health promotion data, rely—in the tradition of the epidemiological model—on illness and risk variables as ultimate criteria in explanation models and outcome evidence (see McQueen, Chapter 4 in this book). In the social epidemiological tradition, it is the social inequality in the "distribution of illness" rather then social inequality in the "production of health" on which public health research and policy seems to be concentrated. It is therefore time to push further with a new focus on the distribution of health rather than disease and to include in our theories explanations on social inequalities in the means for producing health at the societal and the individual level.

2. General Purpose and Aims of the Chapter

Today, health promotion is facing a number of old and new challenges: improving the health of those living in deprived social conditions, strengthening empowerment and participation at all levels of society (see Potvin, Chapter 7), the application of modern tools for health information and life-long-learning (see Balbo, Chapter 8) as well as many more. No one single theory could possibly capture the extensive development required of appropriate concepts and intervention strategies to address all these important areas. However, from a sociological perspective, a theory for health promotion should help meaningfully combine all of these afore-mentioned challenges, including but not limited to the socio-economic and social-cultural factors that constitute health (Kickbusch, 1986). Thus, there is a need for contemporary health promotion theory to explain the interdependence of socio-structural and behavioural factors in the everyday production and maintenance of health.

This chapter presents a theoretical exploration into the question as to what degree the unequal distribution of cultural resources such as values, norms and behavioural patterns, contributes to the persisting social inequalities in population health. More specifically, the chapter looks to particular cultural resources, namely those that can be accumulated, invested and transformed for the sake of health gains and social distinction, or, in other words, it examines cultural resources in their function as a particular form of capital in the production of health and the reproduction of social inequality. Focusing upon that particular part in the production of health that is taking place in people's everyday life, it is argued that cultural capital is one of the most fundamental and socially stratified resources for health in modernity.

The present chapter focuses upon the work of Pierre Bourdieu (Lane, 2000; Fowler, 1997) and his concept of cultural capital. A number of particular features in Bourdieu's approach make it especially useful for applications to current public health and health promotion theory and practice.

1. Bourdieu's theory is based upon a comprehensive theoretical perspective that integrates cultural processes of social differentiation into the broader systems of unequal distribution of life chances. For an emerging theory of health promotion it provides a new and more comprehensive approach to linking social structure with people's cultural resources and behavioural patterns

2. By emphasizing the determining role of social conditions for the cultural pat-terning of behaviours such as eating habits, physical activity etc., Bourdieu takes us beyond the expressive features of health lifestyles and shows how patterns of perceptions, values, norms and behaviours are developed according to particular socio-economic and socio-cultural living conditions. His explanations account for structural constrains, yet also for individual variation and change in perceptions and behaviours, thus reaching beyond simple structural determinism.

3. As Bourdieu's approach integrates different levels of analysis, his work be-comes a particularly useful venue into health promotion issues, that typically link individual behaviour to different levels of collectivity incl. families, peer groups, communities etc.

4. Bourdieu's theory development often links back to "real world experiences" which appear to make his theoretical insights more readily applicable to practical health promotion.

The present chapter pursues three more specific aims.

Firstly, it provides an introduction to Bourdieu's cultural capital theory. This introduction is selective and focussed upon aspects relevant to issues in current health promotion. Despite its selective character it hopes to demonstrate the im-portance of cultural capital to a critical understanding of the production of health.

Through this introduction, this chapter seeks to contribute to a better understanding of the social gap in health and, particularly, of such socio-cultural processes and patterns through which social inequalities are transformed into health inequalities.

Secondly, this chapter aims to lay the foundation for linking the concept of cultural capital to applied issues of modern health promotion. From its perspective of cultural capital theory, it provides an opportunity to re-examine practical intervention approaches in health promotion, and thus address in a new light key issues in public health. Employing two examples of health literacy and health lifestyles, this chapter will show that health promotion measures—besides their health enhancing effects—are also to be understood as modes of the continuous (re-) production of social inequality.

Thirdly, applying basic insights derived from Bourdieu's theory of cultural capital, this chapter offers new light on the current institutionalization process of health promotion. Some critical reflections are provided, emphasizing the need for health promotion to increase its cultural capital in the struggle over resources and power in the health sector.

3. On the Role of Capital for Social Inequality in Health

In public health and particularly in health promotion, the social and cultural conditions of health are key issues in understanding social inequality in health. What are the structural and behavioural conditions necessary for high levels of population health? How are the resources for the production of health distributed across the social strata? Who gains from what kind of investment in good health? Such questions imply issues of investment and return, conflict and power and as such directly relate to basic principles of capital theory. In its most general definition the term "capital" refers to those resources that are generated by labour (e.g. money) including material resources that can be directly transformed into money, e.g. property, financial assets, stocks. Capital resources can be used in the exchange of goods and values or for investments and accumulation of more or other resources. Indeed, since its early days public health research has studied the effects of economic and material resources on health and health care. Over the previous century, social epidemiology has gathered substantial evidence that describes the associations between income or other forms of economic capital and mortality and morbidity using data from different levels of analysis such as individual, community, regional and national. However, despite ample descriptive evidence rather little understanding has been developed accounting for the socio-cultural processes that link the unequal distribution of capital to the social gradients in health (Krieger, 2003).

Moreover, today economic thinking is of increasing importance in health services research and practice and in health promotion. Its focus is on issues of investment in and consumption of health care services and health promotion measures. In both of these two public health areas, theories of market principles are increasingly applied to study and understand the allocation of resources, effectiveness and efficiency of investments etc. Economic approaches to the study of health promotion generally emphasize structural and material conditions. In contrast, sociological thinking in public health often applies to issues centred on non-material aspects in the production and distribution of health such as psycho-social stress, health behaviours, social support systems, norms and values. On these later issues, emphasis is often placed on the role of the actor and his/her socio-cultural context. Thus, two research approaches seem to prevail that focus either on the economic, often material conditions *or* the social-cultural processes of health production and distribution.

As it has been indicated above, capital theories may enhance our understanding of conflict processes such as the struggle over scarce resources and the unequal distribution of power. Compared to other discourses in the health sector (e.g. doctor-patient relationships, rationing of medical services), in health promotion, power issues are less often made explicit. However, there is some discussion on power issues, e.g. on the influence of the medical model in health promotion (WHO Ottawa Charter, 1986) or on conflicting financial interests in applied fields such as work site health promotion etc. When it comes to the unequal distribution of material resources for health, e.g. working and housing conditions, minimum wages etc., power issues are more or less obvious. Cultural resources for health, in contrast, are not often discussed in terms of power issues. They are mostly and often only implicitly considered matters of free choice, individual taste, and consumer preferences. However, socio-cultural resources for health are often also a matter of conflict and power, social inclusion and exclusion. For instance, which (health) consumer patterns are considered appropriate? Who defines, who sets the normative standards when it comes to "proper" lifestyles and health behaviours? What sanctions apply or what benefits are available as a consequence of (not) meeting normative health goals? Those questions indicate that the chances for defining normative health standards, acting in accordance with them as well as the likelihood of benefits are unequally distributed in and across different population groups. Therefore, what is needed today are theories that help to detect and understand the conflictual processes in the promotion of the public's health.

3.1. Economic, Social, and Cultural Capital

In the 1980s a new theory was proposed by Pierre Bourdieu (Lane, 2000; Fowler, 1997), that focused upon the interplay between material and non-material capital as the centre of a comprehensive analysis for social inequality, social stratification and unequal distribution of power. It is perhaps one of Bourdieu's most important contributions that he was able to demonstrate, that the economy of a society reaches far beyond the so-called economic market of that society and thus cannot be fully understood only in terms of classical concepts of economic capital alone, such as property, labour, etc. Bourdieu shows that virtually all areas of society are a part of that economy, constantly contributing to the production and re-production of life chances and opportunities and impacting the unequal distribution of power. More specifically, Bourdieu's work illustrates that, besides economic capital, other

TABLE 5.1. Three types of capital

Types of capital	Basic distinction	Mayor currency	Indicators
Economic	Monetary success versus failure	Money	Economic status
Social	Member versus non-member	Social contacts and connections	Membership
Cultural	Recognition versus indifference	Prestige Knowledge	Reputation, education

Adopted from Anheier, Gerhards & Romo (1995)[1].

forms of capital are also critical to understanding the complex processes of social differentiation in modern societies. Bourdieu distinguishes basically three types of capital: economic, social and cultural. Table 5.1 provides an overview of the types of capital and some of their distinct features.

Bourdieu argues for a primary importance of economic capital for matters of social stratification[2] but stresses that the different types of capital are not independent of each other.

While the role of economic capital (e.g. income) has been studied for a long time in various public health disciplines, cultural capital has thus far been given less attention.[3]

Thus, what appears to be missing in public health and health promotion today, is a more comprehensive theoretical frame that helps us to understand the interplay between the different forms of capital and their role in the production of population health. With contemporary trends in modern societies such as the expanding territories of health, increasing cultural diversity etc. (see McQueen & Kickbusch Introduction) there is a clear need to develop a better understanding of the role of

---

[1] Table 1 has been adopted from Anheier et al. (1995) in different ways:

1. A fourth form of capital (symbolic-cultural) was omitted as it has no central relevance for the present application to health promotion.
2. Departing from the table proposed by Anheier et al. here (and in the following text) we use the term "types" of capital while referring to those particular forms of capital (economic, social, cultural) that provide the most basic forms in Bourdieu's approach (see also footnote on page 13).
3. Focusing upon cultural capital, "knowledge" was added here as a "currency" that is linked to social recognition and education and plays an important role in the production of health through health literacy (see Section 2 in this chapter.)

[2] It can also be argued that the centrality of economic capital might depend upon the basic level of affluence of a given society. In other words, in (sub-) populations in which there is a comparatively high level of economic capital, other types of capital, such as social or cultural capital, may gain in relative importance.

[3] Since the 1990s social capital has received considerable attention in public health research (e.g. Hawe & Shiell, 2000; Kawachi, 2001). However, focusing upon the role of cultural capital, the present chapter does not examine social capital explicitly. Still, it is selectively referred to in health promotion examples on the interplay between different types of capital.

cultural resources in the unequal distribution of health chances and opportunities in society and show how health promotion can improve its policies and actions by taking advantage of that improved knowledge.

3.2. Capital, Habitus, and Field

Bourdieu's larger focus is on the question of "how individuals' routine practices are influenced by the external structure of their social world and how these practices, in turn, contribute to the maintenance of that structure" (Cockerham, Rütten & Abel, 1997; see also Jenkins, 2002). In order to explore the role of cultural capital in this interplay between structures and practice a brief reference to three particular key concepts in Bourdieu's approach appears mandatory. Such key concepts are Habitus, Capital and Field.

Habitus is defined by Bourdieu (1990, p. 52)... "as systems of durable, transposable dispositions, structures predisposed to operate as structuring structures, that is, as principles which generate and organize practices and representations that can be objectively adapted to their outcomes without presupposing a conscious aiming at ends or an express mastery of the operations necessary in order to attain them." Habitus links objective social conditions to people's behaviours and often finds its expression in particular lifestyles, including health lifestyles (Cockerham, Rütten & Abel, 1997). In Bourdieu's theory, habitus is the central concept at the interface between the individual and its socially structured environment. As such habitus is a key element in the explanation of social inequality, its dynamics and patterns of reproduction.

Capital, for Bourdieu remains a concept absolutely essential "to account for the structure and functioning of the social world" (1986, p. 242). He therefore, aims to reintroduce "capital in all its forms and not solely in the one form recognized by economic theory"(1986, p. 242). In this theory, capital includes both material and non-material resources that determine an actor's freedom of action and his or her chances for profit in a particular social field. (Schwingel, 2003, p. 83). As previously mentioned above (see Table 5.1), Bourdieu (1986) distinguishes between three general types of capital. *Economic capital* comprises income, property and other financial assets. When applied to health issues, economic capital in the form of money is needed to buy e.g. health promoting goods or healthy foods. Economic capital is often also essential for improving the pre-conditions for health behaviours, e.g. paying for physical activity classes or through the opportunity to employ somebody to do the housework for the sake of own personal time for health promoting activities *social capital* is. In Bourdieu's understanding, "the sum of the actual and potential resources that can be mobilized through membership in social networks of actors and organizations" (Anheier, Gerhards & Romo, 1995, p. 862). In its relevance for health issues, social capital is for instance often used in community action in attempts to mobilize policy makers to allocate resources for a certain cause, such as the development of a health promoting community infrastructure. *Cultural capital*, finally, refers to such resources that are related to differentiated value systems. This type of capital becomes effective and finds its expressions in personal dispositions and habits (incorporated cultural capital), in the form of educational titles that grant a person a certain social prestige and power (institutionalized cultural capital) or in the form of knowledge and tradition stored in material form such as in books, machines etc. (objective cultural capital). Some specific examples for cultural capital linked to current issues in public health would be: people's health lifestyle preferences (incorporated cultural capital); educational status (institutionalized cultural capital); health guidebooks or health promotion facilities readily accessible (objective cultural capital).

Fields, according to Bourdieu, are mapped out by patterns of (power-) relations among actors that share a common aim or vested interest (e.g. providing health services) and that usually compete with each other over resources or in defining need and supply (Martin, 2003). Bourdieu in his work refers to different fields and sub-fields such as the field of religion, the field of culture etc but does not mention the health sector.[4] However, while he is somewhat cursory in his distinctions between fields and sub-fields in his concept, it is the power relations among the actors that are of primary importance in defining a field. Furthermore, he argues that the content of the different forms of capital depend upon the field to which it is to be applied.

Habitus, capital and field relate to each other as: $(\mathbf{H} \times \mathbf{C}) + \mathbf{F} = \mathbf{P}$. Bourdieu summarizes his thinking with this formula and explains **P**raxis (i.e. the structured functioning of society) as the product of the interplay between **H**abitus and **C**apital, with the interaction of these two differently patterned in specific social **F**ields. As indicated above, the habitus links the perceptions and behaviours of the people to their objective living conditions. It does so according to the types and amounts of capital available to the actors. The interaction of capital and habitus is crucial, yet it may follow different patterns according to the distinct social fields in which it is operating (Bourdieu, 1986; Schwingel, 2003).

The following application of cultural capital theory to issues of social inequality in health promotion relates to these key concepts as follows: Firstly, the present chapter defines health relevant cultural capital as determined by the quantity and quality of available socio-cultural resources that increase the range of the choices for healthy behaviours and improve the chances for changing those living conditions that significantly impact on one's own health or the health of others. Secondly,

---

[4] Health might also be understood as a field in Bourdieu's sense for several of its characteristics: The dealing with health in everyday life is a reflection of fundamental social stratification processes and under the current conditions of modernity, it has also assumed the function of a means of social differentiation (e.g. in the forms of health lifestyles). Moreover, health promotion has become a field of normative struggles over who defines what is appropriate, who follows or is supposed to or expected to follow certain health rules and body regiments. Also, like in other fields, issues of agenda setting and allocation of resources are crucial in public health and health promotion. And certainly the health sector in general has become an economical market of rapidly growing size in which investments and profit margins on the one side and unequal means of consumption and chances to benefit on the other are constituent elements.

States of Cultural Capital	Indicators of Cultural Capital
Incorporated Cultural Capital	social and technical knowledge and skills perceptions, values, behaviours . . .
Objectivized Cultural Capital	books, technical tools, pieces of art . . .
Institutionalized Cultural Capital	educational degrees, status ascription, professional titles . . .

FIGURE 5.1. Indicators of cultural capital.

it follows up on Bourdieu's distinct insights introduced above: cultural, economic and social capital and habitus are key factors for social distinction and patterns of social inequality in the health sector. The chapter sets out to demonstrate the general applicability of both arguments to health promotion measures by referring to health lifestyles and health literacy as two practical examples. Thirdly, it introduces the argument that, particularly in health promotion it is cultural capital that is of pertinent importance for the production and re-production of health inequalities.

The present chapter's focus is on cultural capital as that particular part that, when compared to economical or social capital, has so far been given rather little attention. It does so on the premise that in modern affluent societies, where a basic standard of living secures the survival (incl. basic medical care) for almost all of its members, the relative importance of non-material resources for health and well-being increases. Moreover, under conditions of modernity such as the widening of consumer choices for many and the increasing importance of information processing for a successful management of everyday life, the role of cultural factors for the production of good health is ever increasing.

4. Cultural Capital: An Introduction

According to Bourdieu (1986) cultural capital has its own specific logic that is perhaps clearest in its contrast to the logic of economic capital. Neither its meanings nor its operational categories can be reduced to or substituted by those of economic capital. Fundamentally, Bourdieu distinguishes three states of cultural capital: incorporated, objectivized, and institutionalized cultural capital.[5]

The indicators depicted in Fig. 5.1 are *cultural factors* in so far as they do carry a particular meaning based on systems of social values and norms. At the same time, these factors can be understood as *capital factors* under the condition that

---

[5] There appears to be no consistent use of terminology when it comes to a differentiation of the various kinds of capital in Bourdieu's work. In the following the term "forms" is used in its generic application as the most general concept referring to all types and states of capital. The term "types" is used to distinguish between economical, social and cultural capital. Finally, "states" is used to differentiate sub-categories of cultural capital.

they are productive elements of a society's broader system of social distinction, stratification and unequal distribution of power. For instance, a book or a certain piece of art becomes a fact and factor of cultural capital if the possession of that object is socially linked to a certain value judgement *and* this cultural differentiation contributes to social inequality with respect to prestige and power.

4.1. Incorporated Cultural Capital

Incorporated cultural capital comprises all skills and knowledge of every day practise that can be acquired by "culture". Perhaps closest to what Bourdieu means here by the French term "culture" is a rather broad understanding of education (the German term here is "Bildung") which embraces all forms of learning not only acquiring knowledge but also learning how to behave properly, how to make sense of the world etc. Thus, perceptions, skills and knowledge can be understood as cultural resources that are virtually stored inside the individual human body, and collectively within a given society, subcultures, etc. Such resources are acquired through a social class-specific psycho-social learning process making the incorporation of those resources a lifelong process of capital acquisition. Respective perceptions and behaviours are applied and practised in all social interactions and as such they become daily routines. In contrast to economic capital, incorporated cultural capital is ultimately and profoundly tied to the human body and consequently to a person him- or herself. By being incorporated inside the body in this particular form, cultural capital as such becomes almost entirely invisible. Becoming virtually a part of the body, this state of cultural capital is closely linked to the biological conditions and uniqueness of the actor (Bourdieu, 1986, p. 245).[6]

Incorporated cultural capital has to be personally acquired and the necessary learning processes cannot be delegated. The fact that this investment has to be made by the same person who wants to use the resulting capital indicates that the options and means for accumulation of incorporated cultural capital are limited. It further means that the main source needed to obtain this state of cultural capital is "time", more specifically personal time. Bourdieu concludes from this later observation that the duration of education might be the "least in-accurate" measure of incorporated cultural capital (Bourdieu, 1986. p. 244). Yet, he also stresses that a measure of "time of education" would have to include all stages and forms of lifelong learning including family education, peer group socialization, work environment experience etc.; certainly not just years of schooling. Moreover, as Bourdieu indicates, there is also "negative" incorporated cultural capital: perceptions, skills and behavioural patterns that are properly learned in

---

[6] When it comes to issues of health, not only social but also the biological resources need to be considered. On the later Bourdieu only briefly mentions the links of incorporated cultural capital to the biological system and indicates a significant role of the biological limits and abilities of the social actor (Bourdieu, 1986 p. 245). However, he does not elaborate on this aspect, which would appear, however, particularly important in public health and health promotion and practices.

one particular context or social field might not be appropriate in other contexts or fields. In this case they become a "debit" and may even need additional time to "un-learn".

Incorporated cultural capital needs, beside personal time, also "affection" as its acquisition depends not only on external conditions but also on an interest in the investment in and personal benefits from cultural capital; for example, an affection for higher education and the motivation to invest in educational degrees. The "cultural game" (Schwingel, 2003) in the area of educational inequality also includes that one has to accept and play by the rules of that game. For French society Bourdieu's observes, for example, a normative denial of a direct material interest behind the investment in incorporated cultural capital. This rule of a normative denial of a personal profit expectation plus the "invisibility" of this state of cultural capital (because of its incorporation) are two decisive factors in incorporated cultural capital. Both account for the fact that incorporated cultural capital is not as readily observable than most other forms of capital. As such it becomes, according to Bourdieu, the "best hidden form" of capital (Bourdieu, 1986, p. 246).

Despite the fact that incorporated cultural capital is much less visible than other states of cultural capital, it plays a crucial role in the exchanges of the different forms of capital. The role of incorporated cultural capital is apparent in its links to the two other states of cultural capital namely objectivized and institutionalized cultural capital (see. Fig. 5.1 above): objects of cultural capital like books or tools can only be used as productive resources on the condition that an actor's incorporated cultural capital is sufficient e.g. for understanding the facts and knowledge that are provided in such books, sufficient for using the tools etc. Likewise, institutionalized cultural capital (e.g. formal educational degrees) can normally only be obtained on the basis of sufficient incorporated cultural capital.

4.2. Objectivized Cultural Capital

In its objectivized state, cultural capital comprises books, paintings, machines, technical tools etc. These objects can be seen as material forms and representation of knowledge and meaning developed and accumulated over time in a given society and particular sub-cultures. Its cultural meaning makes it different from economic capital which, in the form of money, has a much more universal meaning and a broader general utility. Still, in its object form cultural capital is in some ways close to economic capital in that its material forms (books, paintings, cars etc.) are transferable across owners or users. However, objectivized cultural capital has its own rules of transformation (Bourdieu, 1986). Transferable is only the object itself, not the ability or competence of using or applying it as a resource beyond its economic trading use. In other words, not readily transferable are the culturally learned abilities, for instance to read and understand a particular book or to enjoy a certain piece of art. The qualitative meaning and the utility value of objectivized cultural capital is dependent upon the incorporated cultural capital of the owner or user.

4.3. Institutionalized Cultural Capital

According to Bourdieu, cultural capital is institutionalized mostly via educational degrees. Such degrees allow the formalized use of incorporated cultural capital. Reaching beyond the mere ability to understand certain phenomena, the particular function and meaning of institutionalized cultural capital is in the formal legitimization and social recognition of incorporated cultural capital. In other words, institutionalized cultural capital (e.g. educational degrees) functions as the formal mode of social recognition of particular forms of cognitive abilities or practical skills and competence. As such it provides wide social acceptance of that competence and boosters the credibility of a certain product or message presented by that actor. Furthermore, as institutionalized cultural capital (e.g. an academic degree) is linked to the actor him/herself, it also increases the social status of the "carrier" of that competence. It also "entitles" the actor to behave according to his or her degree. Consider for example, the case of an autodidact who is missing any educational degree. His or her chances of finding acceptance in a community initiative, having others following his/her advice, getting a high-level job etc., are likely to be reduced than those of somebody carrying a formally "authorized" and "authorizing" academic degree.

While incorporated capital is the state of cultural capital that is most hidden, objectivized cultural capital is the most visible as it evolves in material form. However, when it comes to the processes of how cultural capital works, it is institutionalized cultural capital that is perhaps the most recognizable. As the example of the relevance of formal educational degrees demonstrates, this third state of cultural capital can be understood as a particular mode of status differentiation that is not only highly visible but has also become widely accepted as a determining factor of social stratification in modern societies.

4.4. Interdependence Among the Three States of Cultural Capital

As it has been indicated above, the three states of cultural capital are intertwined. In fact, one might argue that the three forms are more or less mutually dependent (see Figure 5.2). It therefore appears crucial to explore theoretically and empirically the links between the three states of cultural capital in terms of bi- or trilateral dependencies. Moreover, it is also important to understand more fully the recursive transformative processes among the three states of cultural capital. Examples can be used to illustrate these transformative processes. For instance, objectivized cultural capital (e.g. books) is used to acquire or increase personal knowledge. During a necessary personal learning process cultural capital is obtained by an actor through an active transformation of objectivized cultural capital (possession of books) into its incorporated state (internalized knowledge). The resulting new resource, namely knowledge, will add to the actor's general intellectual abilities and skills that could be eventually retransformed through the creation of new

FIGURE 5.2. Three states of cultural capital.

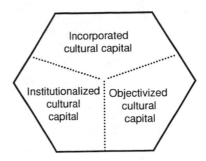

objects of cultural capital, e.g. designing new tools, writing a textbook. In this case incorporated cultural capital is being retransformed from its incorporated state (personal knowledge) into objectivized cultural capital (a textbook). Writing a textbook is likely to promote one's professional career perhaps by obtaining a higher academic degree. In that case objectivized cultural capital is applied and transformed into institutionalized cultural capital.

4.5. Interdependence Among the Three Types of Capital

The three states of cultural capital explored here are mutually dependent and evolved in a complex transformation process. Similar principles can be observed when it comes to the interplay between the broader forms, meaning between the three types of capital, namely economic, social and cultural capital. A minimum asset or stock of each type of capital is required for a successful participation in the game of social distinction. Of central importance yet, less apparent is the fact that capital can and often ought to be transformed from one type to the other. For example, the amount of educational time that is provided to children by their parents is well dependent on the financial situation and economic capital available in the family. If it is possible to provide extensive time of schooling and perhaps directly invest in extra (mostly expensive) learning support (e.g. for exam preparation—something that has become quite common in school careers in many Western societies) economic capital is transformed into cultural capital. Through institutionalized cultural capital—in the most usual cases educational degrees earned—this cultural resource is later retransformed into economical capital e.g. via better paid jobs for those with higher degrees. There could be many more examples that demonstrate the relevance of such interdependence and transformation processes at all levels of society ranging from individual action to competitions among whole institutions (see paragraph V "Epilogue").

According to Bourdieu these transformative processes within and between the different forms (i.e. types and states) of capital determine the unequal distribution of resources and power in most modern societies. One then can argue that in its most radical application, the interplay between the different forms of capital underlie all social differentiations in modern Western societies.

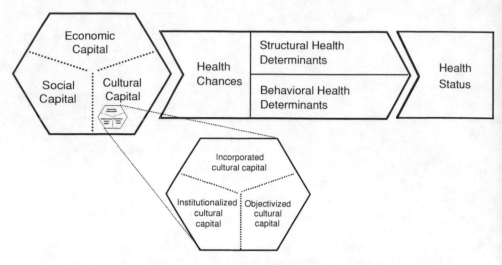

FIGURE 5.3. Capital interaction and health.

Applying Bourdieu's theory to inequalities in health one can argue that the interplay between different types and states of capital provides the core to the processes that structure the unequal distribution of health. Figure 5.3 illustrates how the interplay between different forms of capital provide foundation to the production and social distribution of health.

The dotted lines in the graph emphasize the interaction and transformations along the different forms of capital. According to empirical evidence available today, health-effective economic capital comprises resources such as income, housing, private health insurance plans and other tangible material resources. Respectively social capital entails social support and trust, while cultural capital includes among other factors education, values and social norms. Unequally distributed supply of economic, social and cultural capital affects health chances and opportunities at the collective and individual level. Health chances are understood here as structurally anchored probabilities for good health. They comprise structural health determinants (e.g. access to medical care and health promotion) and behavioural determinants (e.g. risk or health enhancing behaviour patterns) that increase or decrease the likelihood of good health. The processes indicated in this figure should not be seen as a completely linear relationship but include also recursive links, e.g. from health back to the chances of acquiring different forms of capital. While—from a behavioural perspective—such processes may also apply to individuals, from Bourdieu's perspective, it is meant to primarily describe collective patterns typical for particular socio-economic segments or social-cultural groups of any given society.

At this point we can summarize and conclude that cultural capital evolves in its three interdependent states of incorporated, objectivized and institutionalized cultural capital. Cultural capital is a non-replaceable factor and function in a broader system of social stratification, capital accumulation and transformation. This broader system regulates the un-equal distribution of life chances and power on the basis of a continuous interplay between economical, social and cultural capital. Cultural capital plays a particular role in this broader system and as such, has its own distinct logic and categories. The logic of incorporated cultural capital rests on four particular features: 1. it is bound to the body 2. it needs personal time to be obtained and incorporated 3. its acquisition and application needs affection for and interest in the cultural game 4. it is based on specific rules of the cultural game.

5. Cultural Capital: Applications in Health Promotion Practice

The production and distribution of health depends upon the complex interplay of structural and behavioural factors. Theoretical approaches in health promotion therefore need to address the interaction between structure and agency (e.g. Cockerham, 2005). Social-cultural conditions appear of utmost importance for this interaction. Today's widening of lifestyle choices, new modes of learning and communicating, new ways to search for health information etc. provide particular social-cultural conditions that directly affect people's health, health chances and opportunities.

At this point, a crucial question for health promotion arises: to whom do these particular social and technical innovations apply and who benefits (most) from opportunities arising from modern social change? One should ask whether the widening of health related lifestyle options or improved access to health information apply to the same degree for the young and the old, the rich and the poor, the high and the low educated.

Such issues pose major challenges in health promotion today. In addressing the questions that arise from these issues, an application of Bourdieu's theory of cultural capital is fruitful in several ways. First, it shifts our attention from the description of social inequalities in health to the explanation of how those inequalities are produced and re-produced. Secondly, it shows how the social structures shape the perceptions and actions of the individuals and vice versa. Thirdly, by emphasizing the central importance of the incorporation of cultural capital it widens our understanding of the role of the human body in the social stratification of health. Thus, the cultural capital approach is helpful to illustrate how sociological theory can be applied to better understand current issues health promotion practice. But also, applying this particular theory to existing intervention models can provide a new channel through which critical assessment and self-reflexive feedback from field experts can feed back into the discourse on theory in health promotion (see Potvin, Chapter 7 in this book).

In the present chapter the perspective of cultural capital theory is applied to look critically at health lifestyles and health literacy as two popular approaches in current health promotion. This application starts with a proposition that defines the improvement of health chances as the principal goal of modern health promotion and, consequently, argues that health promotion interventions need to be assessed, theoretically and empirically, as for their role in improving health chances of the population and specific target groups. A critical assessment would have to include the impact of interventions on improving health chances, in particular in those subpopulations with a lack of social resources. It also has to address the risk of adverse effects that could lead to a widening of the social gap in health chances. It will be argued here that health literacy and health lifestyle are specific forms of incorporated cultural capital and as such they are both: social-cultural resources for health and at the same time, dynamic modes of social inequalities in the production and distribution of health.

5.1. Example 1: Health Literacy

5.1.1. Health Literacy and Health Promotion

Having been applied earlier in approaches to patient information/compliance (Eysenbach, Powell, Kuss & Sa, 2002; Davis & Wolf, 2004) or in community development (Freire, 1985), health literacy has been introduced to health promotion as late as the 1980s. WHO (Nutbeam, 1998) has defined health literacy as reaching beyond basic skills of reading and understanding health information to include . . . "the cognitive and social skills which determine the motivation and ability of individuals to gain access to, understand and use information in ways which promote and maintain good health".

Nutbeam (2000) suggests a model that distinguishes three levels of health literacy: On the lowest level, *functional health literacy* refers to the basic understanding of factual health information. On the second level more advanced cognitive and literacy skills join with social skills to improve an individual's personal capacity for interactive communication (*interactive health literacy*). On the most advanced level *critical health literacy* allows the individual to critically analyse and apply health information for the sake of greater control over life events and situations.

Some of the approaches to health literacy have been criticized for their too individualistic focus emphasizing the socio-cultural context in which health literacy is learned, as well as the varying meanings of health literacy in different social settings (Kickbusch, 2001).

More recently Abel and Bruhin (2003) have defined health literacy as the knowledge-based competency for health promoting behaviours including the social engagement in broader health issues. In their approach "knowledge" is understood primarily as "lay" knowledge relating to health and illness experiences in everyday life. Such knowledge is learned through family and peer group cultures, primary and secondary education as well as less formal ways of learning via new media access (Abel & Bruhin, 2003). Thus health literacy includes access to, as well as understanding and critical assessment of, health information. Adequate health literacy not only supports personal health management but also increases the chances of changing health-relevant living conditions. Most generally speaking, when applied to health promotion practice, health literacy means to understand the conditions that determine health and to know how to change them.

Traditionally, health education and health promotion have been aimed at improving health literacy of individuals and populations by teaching or providing information on specific health matters. However, the development of health literacy is not independent of the general level of primary literacy in any given population. Moreover, low primary literacy affects people's health not only via insufficient means to understand health messages but also by the chances for social or cultural participation in general. Given the increasing importance of health issues in modern societies (see McQueen & Kickbusch, Introduction in this book) these later observations indicate a prominent role of health literacy in a broader system of the unequal distribution of health opportunities.

5.1.2. Health Literacy as a Socio-Cultural Resource for Health

From the theoretical perspective of cultural capital, health literacy is a resource for increasing the chances for health gains. There are various ways in which advanced health literacy can improve one's health chances. Health literacy as incorporated cultural capital comprises values and norms that affect people's perceptions of health and illness. Moreover, a considerable stock of health literacy is necessary to relate, in a meaningful way, public health messages (e.g. health promotion recommendations) to one's own life situation, to find means and ways of realising behavioural change, to engage in community action to improve health promoting neighbourhood infrastructures etc.

As these examples indicate, health literacy can also promote the effective use of different forms of capital such as objectivized cultural capital (e.g. books) or social capital, for instance by opening the way into neighbourhood networks or self-help groups. An advanced degree of health literacy can thus be helpful not only for improving directly one's health chances but also contributes to the chances of social participation and the more effective use of different forms of capital.

5.1.3. Health Literacy and the (Re-)Production of Social Inequality in Health

Health promotion measures have been suggested to improve health literacy in the population. Yet, there appears to be less awareness that certain health promotion interventions might increase rather than reduce social inequality in health literacy. This would be the case, if for instance new information technologies for health promotion were not critically assessed for general accessibility and adequate forms of presentation, a case in point being health information on the internet. Current studies have provided critical evidence of a significant "digital divide" in the use of the internet for health information and advice (Davis & Wolf, 2004). Consequently health promotion interventions via health literacy need to take into account that they carry the potential for decreasing as well as the risk of increasing social inequality.

Moreover, the role of health literacy as a mode of the (re-)production of social inequality goes far beyond issues of accessibility to health information. High or low health literacy improves or hampers not only the health choices of individuals and their opportunities for certain health relevant behaviours, but it also promotes shared perceptions of health, attitudes and orientations often typical for different social groups. Moreover, chances to participate in joined action for health and shared decision-making may well depend upon the health knowledge of an individual and his or her ability to communicate and interact with others. Beyond issues of personal interaction, health literacy as cultural capital may support the accumulation of other forms of capital for health. Take the example of a citizen who wants to become involved in health promotion at the community level: he or she, being concerned about a health matter in the neighbourhood might use his/her knowledge to write a letter to the reader's corner of a local newspaper. Depending upon the contents and the readership this may yield social recognition in the neighbourhood and even consecutive social support for further action. Applying his/her cultural capital in this way, may also increase his/her chances of becoming an active member of (other) social or interest groups, contributing to their social capital. The theory of cultural capital would thus explain the double function of health literacy: it emerges as a resource for health and at the same time is functioning as a mode of social inequality.

As indicated above, when it comes to critical health literacy, empowerment plays an important role. If, for instance, health knowledge were increased on the population level only in the sense of "expert advice" to be followed, leaving out measures to improve people's abilities to critically select or assess such (and other) health counselling, health promotion itself would create new dependencies. In order to avoid new forms of paternalism, in which dominance of medical expert advice were substituted by "health promotion expert advice", health literacy interventions should built upon and increase the cultural capital in all its forms, incl. critical health literacy. Health literacy should be seen as a dynamic and reciprocal component in health empowerment. Perceiving health literacy as an embedded form of cultural capital leads to an emphasis of the empowerment component in health promotion interventions. Consequently, health promotion interventions should start with a critical assessment of the cultural capital (not) available in those specific population groups they hope to work with. Also, interventions should focus on those population groups who have less of this particular resource because such interventions would otherwise contribute to rather than reduce social inequality in the chances for good health.

In modern social and cultural conditions health literacy is a basic pre-requisite and vital resource for managing one's personal health, as well as active participation in community-based health action. Countries like Australia, Great Britain and the United States, have recently included health literacy as explicit targets in their national health policies. From the perspective of cultural capital theory, health literacy interventions are basic investments in people's general cultural capital, not only for the sake of better health outcomes but also because of in-creasing chances for social participation and self-directed action. With respect to issues of social stratification, health literacy needs to be promoted for and foremost amongst those population groups that have the least supply of overall literacy and health literacy. To achieve this, it would appear necessary to improve access to traditional (e.g. brochures, posters, promotional materials) as well as more inter-active technological sources (e.g. internet) of health information and develop new and targeted mechanisms for information and dissemination. Beside such basic issues of access, quality of information and the ways in which health informa-tion is presented, is also of great importance (Eysenbach, Powell, Kuss & Sa, 2002; Davis & Wolf, 2004). For both, access and dissemination, one would need to know more about the information seeking behaviours among these targeted populations.

5.2. Example 2: Health Lifestyles

5.2.1. Health Lifestyles and Health Promotion

Like lifestyles in general, health lifestyles seem to gain an ever-increasing impor-tance in modernity (see McQueen & Kickbusch, Introduction in this book). Under conditions of constant change and increasing choices, lifestyles meet utilitarian needs but also help to develop and maintain self-identity and ontological security (Giddens, 1991; Cockerham, Rütten & Abel, 1997). For most, however, lifestyle choices are hardly "free" choices, rather they are limited by restrictions that are more or less obvious to the outside observer (Abel, Cockerham & Niemann, 2000; Frohlich, Corin & Potvin, 2001). Most obvious perhaps are economic limitations (e.g. income) and social norms (e.g. peer group expectations). Beyond such fac-tors, Bourdieu (1984) argues that lifestyle choices are not only constrained but also shaped by the life chances typical for different social classes. In a critical review of different sociological theories of lifestyles Cockerham et al (1997) found that a different focus on either "choice" (most prominent perhaps in the work of Giddens, 1991) or "chance" (strongly emphasized by Bourdieu) is the leading issue in the current discourse on lifestyles in modernity.

On the basis of earlier theoretical analyses we have addressed this central issue and defined health lifestyles accordingly as comprising "... interacting patterns of health related behaviours, orientations and resources adapted by groups of in-dividuals in response to their social, cultural and economic environment" (Abel, Cockerham & Niemann, 2000). The concept of health related lifestyles as de-veloped by Abel and his collaborators (Abel, 1991; Cockerham, Rütten & Abel, 1997; Abel, 2000) includes several characteristics that make it different from ear-lier, mostly risk-factor-oriented lifestyle approaches in social epidemiology: firstly, it integrates behaviours, attitudes and resources as three equally important con-stituent dimensions of health lifestyles. Second, rather than focussing upon either choice *or* chance it stresses in a Weberian tradition (see Abel, 1991) the interplay between the structural pre-conditions (the "givens") of health lifestyles on the one side and the preferences and creative action of the people (choosing different lifestyle elements or patterns) on the other side. In this relationship no strict causality or determinism between individual and structural factors is presumed. Thirdly, it allows one to include different perspectives (scientific or lay) on what qualifies for or what defines an "appropriate" health lifestyle pattern. Fourthly, the definition on which the concept is based does not presume health gains as the decisive motive for change of a particular lifestyle; it acknowledges that health relevant lifestyles can be and often are adopted by individuals or whole population groups for reasons other than health. In other words, certain lifestyles, despite the fact that they may be relevant for health, are practiced habitually, with no deliberate intention towards any specific outcome beyond making ends meet. In fact one might speculate that it is often exactly those lifestyles in precarious social and economic conditions, which have the highest risk of being detrimental to the people's health. However, this does not negate the idea that increasingly health lifestyles today are adopted for reasons of improving one's health, physical appearance or fitness. Drawing upon Bourdieu's theory, one can observe, however, that the interest or incentives for personal investment in health (e.g. by means of lifestyle changes) is socially learned and often part and expression of a broader habitus. Such lifestyles become part of (mostly social class specific) cultural capital and acquire symbolic value. Accordingly, Bourdieu views the human body as "physical capital that is transformed into cultural capital as a consequence of social practices" (Cockerham, Rütten & Abel, 1997).

5.2.2. Health Lifestyle as a Socio-Cultural Resource for Health

Today, there is ample evidence for multi-faceted effects of behavioural and other psycho-social determinants of health, many of which can be understood as integral parts of modern lifestyles (Berkmann & Kawachi, 2000; Blaxter, 1900; Berkmann & Breslow, 1983). However, from a sociological perspective the potentially positive or detrimental effects of health lifestyles reach beyond the health and wellbeing of individuals; indeed, beyond their impact on individual health, socially structured lifestyle patterns are determining factors of collective health (e.g. in families, communities and larger social-cultural milieus) (Frohlich, 1999; Williams, 1995). Certain lifestyles, specifically those typical for some religious groups (a particularly interesting religious group in this respect are the Mormons) are known for their impact on good collective health, which is attributed to their particular patterns of behaviours, norms, systems of social support etc. (Koenig, McCollough & Larson, 2001; Powell, Shahabi & Thoresen, 2003). In that sense lifestyles can be understood as active factors in the production of a collective good, and in this instance, health. Moreover, health lifestyles can become an integral part of collective empowerment processes when behaviours, goals of action and available resources are deliberately selected or rearranged in order to improve structural living conditions (Abel, Cockerham & Niemann, 2000). It seems quite feasible that people would make a commitment for community action a part of their lifestyle, contributing with their engagement to a strengthening and quality improvement of their social environment by actively participating in neighbourhood health actions, such as organizing physical activity programs or movements to reduce traffic and air pollution.

5.2.3. Health Lifestyles and the (Re-) Production of Social Inequality in Health

There is great socio-cultural and social-economical diversity when it comes to health related lifestyles. Research has shown that patterns of health related behaviours, attitudes, and resources are very different in different social classes, subcultures, age- and gender groups (Blaxter, 1990; Abel, Cockerham & Niemann, 2000; Cockerham, 2005). Health lifestyles, like other lifestyles, serve as a means of social distinction and have consequently been discovered and promoted by the consumer industry as profitable markets with consumer goods increasingly shaped to meet the (supposed) health and wellness needs of distinct population groups (see Kickbusch, Chapter 9 in this book). For social theory, however, lifestyle distinctions serve the development and maintenance of self identity in modernity (e.g. Giddens, 1991) but also serve the maintenance of the basic patterns of the unequal distribution of power (Bourdieu, 1984). As Bourdieu (1984) explains, one particular feature of incorporated cultural capital is that actors learn to use symbolic representation of this capital, wherever and whenever it supports their action. For example perhaps most readily observable in the professional world, material objects (e.g. expensive business clothes) or rules of verbal interaction (e.g. conversation styles) are used to qualify and identify oneself as a member and to demonstrate intellectual superiority. In a similar line of argument, healthy lifestyles can be seen as a social practice to promote social identity and create social distinction among members of certain societal groups. As such health lifestyles become part and expression of cultural capital developed and used by certain groups for the sake of socio-cultural distinction and in the struggle over social esteem, privileges and power.

For instance the use of certain specific sports clothes ("sportive outfits") for exercise groups, the knowledge about nutritional facts and the serving of healthy food to guests, referring to health books in personal conversations etc. can be understood as cultural capital applied in the game over social belonging, distinction and status. Moreover, single health lifestyle elements have to match the broader pattern of social distinction. Consistency in the selection of certain lifestyle elements is closely related to capital transformation processes. For instance a certain degree of advanced health literacy (incorporated cultural capital) will influence or guide the selection of different supporting objects or tools such as health guidebooks (objectivized cultural capital). In this example objectivized cultural capital interacts with incorporated cultural capital to not only contribute to a congruent and healthy lifestyle but also to a positioning of those who have more capital to play in the game of social distinction. This process of mutual investment and transformation of different states of cultural capital is even more decisive when other forms of capital (e.g. economic capital) are to be included, e.g. when expensive sporting goods are symbolizing superior financial means and power.

As one can see, understanding health lifestyles beyond their effects on individual health reaches deeper to the roots of a society's basic system of social differentiation. According to such a perspective, health-promoting lifestyles can serve very different functions. While they potentially enhance people's health, they also serve the need for social distinctions, promote self-identity avail a sense of belonging. However, personal body management, the social use of the body, habitus and health lifestyles are part of a social learning and adoption process in which cultural capital plays a decisive role. Cultural capital is necessary to learn and adopt distinct lifestyle patterns that are appropriate to the social, economic and cultural context in which people develop and grow. From a critical structural perspective, different issues of conflict arise when one tries to understand health lifestyles as part of people's cultural capital. For example, which forms of health relevant lifestyles are defined as appropriate? Who develops and promotes such definitions? What are the sanctions applied with respect to proper or deviant health lifestyles? These and similar questions point to the fact that in interventions through a lifestyle approach one automatically deals with issues of social stratification and power.

Derived from the theoretical consideration above, it can be concluded that cultural capital plays a crucial role in the process of the social patterning of lifestyles incl. those relevant for health. Cultural capital allows peoples to select and link different lifestyle elements and combine them into distinct health lifestyle patterns. This process takes place within particular socio-cultural environments and has to be adjusted to the material and non-material options and resources available to them. There are three nexuses within which such interactive linking process can be observed. Within the first nexus, single elements of health lifestyles have to be selected and arranged as complementary to one another (e.g. eating habits must fit physical activity patterns, behaviours have to match with attitudes and individual resources). Second, health lifestyle patterns need to be in accordance with the socio-cultural and social-economic contexts of the actor (e.g. lifestyle patterns emphasizing health and wellness may or may not be appropriate or affordable in certain milieus).

A third but different kind of nexus at which cultural capital plays a decisive role for health lifestyles refers to the additive value and the transformation of the different types of capital, in general, and the different states of cultural capital in particular. One example for the transformation of different types of capital are financial resources (economic capital) invested to buy, use and socially display objects (e.g. sport outfits) that signify proper health behaviours and attitudes (cultural capital). Transformations among different states of cultural capital refer to the interplay of incorporated cultural capital (e.g. health literacy) and objectivized cultural capital (e.g. the use and possession of health books).

Linking cultural capital theory to the concept of health related lifestyles, there are two major lessons to be learned for health promotion: First, health lifestyles are active parts of social stratification systems; and Second, the development, maintenance and change of health lifestyles depend upon the availability of economic, social and cultural resources with the different states of cultural capital playing a crucial role. Both findings could provide new and more appropriate starting points for innovative concepts in health promotion practice. For example, health lifestyles serve the need for social distinction, and do so differently for different social groups. For health promotion measures it is thus important to recognize these varying needs. As a consequence, the promotion of one quasi "universal" health enhancing lifestyle would appear rather inappropriate, as it neglects the different interests in and need for social distinction and identity as well as the different social, economic and cultural resources available to diverse sub-populations. The alternative may lie in approaches that promote and embrace cultural diversity in health relevant lifestyles, respecting and building upon existing capacities, abilities and skills in different intervention groups (see Potvin, Chapter 7 in this book).

6. Summary

This brief discussion on health literacy and health lifestyles was intended to show that the search conditions and consequences of current approaches in health promotion can be better understood within the theoretical context of cultural capital. In particular, when it comes to social inequality, we can observe that cultural capital resources as represented in the two concepts of health literacy and health lifestyles are essential in the production and distribution of health. These resources are, however, unequally distributed across the social classes and the forms of applying available resources for health are diverse in the different social strata. Consequently, it is suggested that health promotion practice should give increased attention to issues of social inequality and cultural capital for health at the early stages of intervention planning.

7. Conclusions: Towards a Theory of Health Promotion and Social Inequality

Social determinants of health have traditionally been the focus of social medicine and social epidemiology. Epidemiological evidence has demonstrated over and over again that traditional and current forms of social inequality are systematically linked to health outcomes. However, even modern social epidemiology is mostly limited to an exploration of the behavioural and structural health determinants (e.g. risk behaviours and income disparities), treating health and illness as the "endogenous" variable. While the findings from social epidemiologic research are of great importance for descriptive accounts of the distribution of health and disease in our populations, such data do not provide answers to the more basic questions on the relationships between social differentiation and health in modern societies. More specifically, it does not afford the opportunity to address conclusively why and how certain behaviours relevant to health outcomes have become normative in certain populations and not in others. On those issues, sociological theory calls for an understanding of health and health promotion as integrated parts of broader systems of social differentiation and inequality.

Bourdieu's theory of social inequality focuses upon the role of the unequal distribution of capital for the (re-) production of privilege and power. The present chapter provides insights derived from Bourdieu's theory of cultural capital to further the understanding of the unequal distribution of resources for health. Emphasizing the interplay of economic, social and cultural aspects of social inequality Bourdieu's approach merges structural and behavioural factors into one coherent theoretical explanation. These aspects appear to be particularly applicable to health promotion as the production and distribution of health typically relate jointly to aspects of economic, social and cultural resources. The interaction of those aspects point to the complex interplay between the structural conditions provided by society and the actions taken (or not) by their members. The goal of this chapter has been to theoretically explore the role that cultural capital plays in the production of health and how the unequal distribution of cultural capital affects the (re) production of social health inequalities.

Today, and despite some shifts in rhetoric, social inequality in population health and health promotion practice persists. Yet, particularly in affluent societies the emergence of new forms of social differentiation has increased the complexity involved in the production and distribution of health. As a consequence, the central challenge for modern public health is to better understand both old and new dimensions of health inequality under the current social, economic and cultural conditions. In that respect, two theoretical propositions can be derived from Bourdieu's theory of cultural capital:

First, a minimal stock not only of economic but also cultural capital is necessary to produce good health and to successfully participate in the cultural game over social distinction. Second, for the acquisition, adequate use and increase of diverse resources relevant to health, the constant exchange and transformation of different forms of capital is a major underlying principle. To give one final example for the pertinence of capital transformation for health, one can look at personal time and income as two distinct resources for health. It appears a rather obvious fact that personal disposable time is a condition for most health enhancing activities. Yet, applying a cultural capital perspective, we can further explain that personal time is required to obtain the knowledge and skills that are needed to realise e.g. a health promoting lifestyle. Health promoting behaviours and attitudes are parts of people's incorporated cultural capital and have to be learned by investing personal time as the learning cannot be delegated or bought. However, depending on the life circumstances, time for investing in cultural capital is often unequally distributed among certain social groups. Also, personal time for investing in one's own health may be obtained e.g. by arranging child day care or by reducing workloads, but only by those who have the financial means to afford this. There are, however, other, non-material conditions such as interest and commitment that are also pre-requisites for engagement in personal or community health promotion. Yet, health related values and attitudes are socially learned, e.g. in the family context or among peers, thus emphasizing again the structural conditions for the acquisition of health-relevant cultural capital. Financial means, on the other hand, are part of one's economic capital, which is in form of income, also known as a resource for health. Financial resources directly affect health e.g. by the simple fact that one can afford living in a safe and healthy environment. Yet, as economic capital they can also be transformed into cultural capital relevant for health e.g. by making advanced school education possible for the children of that family. Although we have here not discussed at any length the role of social capital, it was indicated that financial and cultural resources can both be invested and transformed also into social capital e.g. by becoming a member in certain clubs or interest groups.

WHO's Ottawa Charter (1986) calls for tackling "the inequalities in health produced by the rules and practices of (..these) societies". This chapter hopes to shed light on how Bourdieu's cultural capital theory contributes to a better understanding of these rules and practices. In that respect, the main points from the present theoretical exploration can be summarised as:

1. Cultural capital, besides and along with economic and social capital plays a crucial role in the unequal production and distribution of health;
2. In health promotion, cultural capital is an indispensable factor in the process of constant exchange and transformation of different forms of health relevant capital including economic and social capital. A sufficient stock of each of these types of capital is necessary to allow for and to benefit from a personal investment in health. Beyond health returns, personal investments in certain lifestyles relevant for health, can serve people's need for social distinction and their struggle over privileges and power;
3. Incorporated, institutionalized and objectivized cultural capital are interdependent and mutually beneficial in their effectiveness for improving the health of different social groups and strata;
4. When is comes to health literacy and health lifestyles, it is incorporated cultural capital that plays the most important role in the development and maintenance of values, perceptions and behaviours that serve both the production of good health and social distinction.

The present application of the cultural capital theory to issues of public health provides new insights in the unequal production and distribution of health and places modern health promotion directly in the current discourse of social in-equality under conditions of modernity (see Pelikan, Chapter 6 in this book). On the background of ongoing social change towards increasing individualisa-tion, of rapidly growing knowledge and exchange of ideas and increasing mi-gration it can be projected that most modern societies will experience a drastic increase in cultural diversity. In that process, the task of health promotion is to contribute to social change that reduces health inequality. Understanding the role of cultural capital in the links of social inequality and cultural diversity will soon become a central issue for public health and a major challenge for health promotion.

8. *Epilogue*: Cultural Capital in the Institutionalization of Health Promotion

The main objective of the present chapter was to introduce, in general, the contribution of Bourdieu's cultural capital approach to theory development its health promotion with a focus on issues of social inequality. The basic principles introduced could also be applied to theory development in an institutional perspective. Current attempts to establish health promotion as an institution within the health sector provide another example for an application of capital transformation principles at the structural level. Emerging as a new institution health promotion is entering a field of action in which the struggle over limited societal resources and power includes different interest groups, the strongest perhaps the medical institutions and disciplines.

Today the health services sector can be seen as what Bourdieu calls an "economic field", meaning it is a social space in which different interest groups apply and invest their capital in a game over profits, power and privileges. This game reaches beyond the fight for financial resources; indeed, it includes issues of definitions and classifications of diseases, as well as agenda setting in health policy, medical sciences and public health. Thus, to operate successfully in such an economic field, cultural and social capital are important resources e.g. for agenda setting, networking, communicating and lobbying. The successful application of the different types of capital is one key factor that has allowed today's medical services sector to develop into a "relative autonomous field", with a high degree of differentiated interests, profitable markets, etc.

In contrast, health promotion, since the Ottawa Charter's inauguration, has mainly tried to establish itself in what might be called a cultural field, meaning, by introducing new definitions of health, by focusing on the production and maintenance of health in every day life rather than professional expert intervention, by deliberately linking its actions to particular societal values, such as solidarity and equal opportunities for health, by shifting paradigms towards intersectorial health promoting policies, etc. However, health promotion is lacking a sufficient stock of cultural capital meaning, there is no wide recognition or regard at the population level, nor are there definitive, standardized text books or established and accredited curricula, academic titles etc. Without those cultural factors, there is little chance to increase its autonomy and improve its chances for competition with the medical model of enhancing the public's health. Additionally, health promotion is lacking evidence on its immediate medical, economical and social impacts (e.g.

reducing morbidity, limit health care cost or improving social integration) which further weakens its economic and political relevance and societal legitimization. Predictable benefits, especially profit expectations according to Bourdieu, are essential and decisive factors in an economic field; without which health promotion remains a voluntary and as such may be considered either obsolete or as belonging to the voluntary sector of society.

Given today's intensifying struggle for resources, competition among the public and private players in the health field will continue to increase. Only those interest groups will survive that have sufficient capital to invest in this competition. Moreover, some will gain even more power and resources, namely those players that can rely on the effective transformation of diverse forms of capital. Medicine, as an established and well-organized system has many favourable pre-conditions: its stock of economic, social and cultural capital has historically grown strong and the transformation processes between them work well. For example it has developed the cultural capital necessary to define the health needs and demands of a population, gain support and societal and political acceptance of those definitions and then have the public sector to provide financial resources, administrative structures, and political authorization needed to react and attend to those needs and demands. Cultural capital is applied in a form that allows the invested money to remain within a rather closed system of medical care services. The gains (personal and population health) yielded from the investment of economic capital are highly "valued" by society at both the individual and collective level. As such, reinforced acceptance and support contribute to an increase in medical cultural capital, as is seen by compliance of medical advice or granted expert status even beyond simply issues in medicine per se. An example of this would be health promotion media campaigns: despite the fact that in health promotion, psycho-social expertise (e.g. how to change behaviour patterns etc) is often more relevant than medical expertise, medical doctors are most often present in the media and asked to provide advise to the lay public regarding the importance of lifestyles change. What may appear questionable with respect to issues of substantive expertise, is plausibly explained from the perspective of the cultural capital theory: authority and dominance of those who have a higher level of institutionalized cultural capital (as partly expressed in the academic title of an MD) is a functional part of the game over authority and power in the public health sector.

The importance of institutionalized cultural capital, for example, advanced educational degrees, applies at all levels of society but is perhaps most readily observable in traditionally structured organizations. Highly formalized bureaucracies provide interesting examples of how institutionalized cultural capital has become an integral part of social hierarchies. So that, a second example from the health sector may illustrate how the interaction between different states of cultural capital serves the maintenance of a given hierarchy of professional titles. In leading public health institutions around the world, an increasing number of middle-ranked research positions are filled today with experts from the social sciences. Despite the fact that these experts have no medical background they are often assigned a medical position, meaning, hired as "senior medical scientists". In this case, in order to reach higher senior positions in a large public health institution, social scientists have to deny or give up their professional name and formal disciplinary identity. While the pragmatic reason for this might be that the bureaucracy is too slow to adapt to the cultural shifts in the academic labour market, the consequences are highly relevant to the formal distribution of power within such institutions, as well as for the disciplines at large including the societal "value" of the respective degrees. What may become a gain for the single individual in terms of a personal career can, from a structural perspective, be seen, in general, as a devaluation and denial of the social sciences professions and non-medical paradigms. Integrating and subordinating cultural capital (theoretical or methodological health expertise) from a "foreign" discipline under the formal degree of a medical position and expertise secures or at least supports the maintenance of definitional and distributive power in the health research sector.

Admittedly, one can argue that such examples of the links between cultural capital accumulation and professional dominance present somewhat crude oversimplifications and may require a more differentiated analysis. Still, the two examples aforementioned may serve to denote the basic principles at play in the struggle for power in the health sector. It also points to the consequences for health promotion when it tries to enter the health sector as an institutional player struggling for professional acceptance and trying to compete over public resources.

If competition for public resources in the health sector continues to increase, then the role of cultural and economic capital will become even more crucial for health promotion to survive. Today health promotion's stock of economic capital is rather poor, and there is little to gain with a rather hypothetical argument of its cost saving effects. As for its cultural capital, health promotion, at least since Ottawa, has tried to increase its definitional power by proposing positive definitions of health, emphasizing lay health resources and empowerment as the priority means to improve population health. However, these attempts have been only moderately successful and are recently challenged by increasing pressure towards new forms of outcome evidence, whose principles are defined, by the medical model of health and disease. With regard to its investment in cultural capital, health promotion has so far made its greatest efforts in the area of incorporated cultural capital, for instance by trying to improve individual health knowledge with the aim of changing people's behaviours, attitudes, values, and norms. With respect to objectivized cultural capital (text books etc) health promotion is advancing slowly. Yet, its stock of objectivized cultural capital is still marginal when compared to other sectors such as medical care. Institutionalized cultural capital of health promotion is also only beginning to grow (e.g. national and international Health Promotion Foundations, academic training programs and positions, educational degrees etc).

As Bourdieu explains at length in his general theory of capital and power, from which this chapter provides a few examples, the transformation processes between economic, social and cultural capital play a crucial role in the struggle over resources and power in distinct fields. Applied to the health sector, one can argue that health promotion today does yet not have sufficient capital to play in the currently intensifying game over resources in the health sector. A sufficient stock of different forms of capital would, however, be necessary in order to make the crucial transformation and exchange processes between economical, social and cultural resources possible. These factors and processes will become more important the more the health sector is transformed into a health market where the rules of the game are dictated by market economies and their specific input and outcome criteria.

While more scrutinized explorations on these issues are needed, there are two major implications to be drawn from this first and brief application of Bourdieu's cultural capital to the issue of an institutionalization of health promotion. First, in order to develop into a relative autonomous field in an increasingly diverse health sector, health promotion has to increase its cultural capital. Key elements for this would be the development of genuine definitions of its subject matter, the application of unique intervention methods and evaluation techniques and the promotion of distinct professional programs and degrees. While building up strong cultural capital appears mandatory, it will not proof sufficient to gain the status of a major public health institution. Thus (and second) in order to survive the increasing competition for public resources or even grow in influence and institutional power, health promotion also needs to build up a sufficient stock of economic and social capital. It is only when the transformation processes between its three types of capital start to accelerate that health promotion, as an institution, will be able to establish itself as a powerful player in the health sector.

References

Abel, T. (1991). Measuring health lifestyles in a comparative analysis: theoretical issues and empirical findings. *Social Science and Medicine, 32*, 899–908.

Abel, T., & Bruhin, E. (2003). Health literacy/Wissensbasierte Gesundheitskompetenz. In Bundeszentrale für gesundheitliche Aufklärung (Ed.), *Leitbegriffe der Gesundheitsförderung: Glossar zu Konzepten, Strategien und Methoden in der Gesundheitsförderung* (pp. 128–131). Schwabenheim: Peter Sabo.

Abel, T., Cockerham, W. C., & Niemann, S. (2000). A critical approach to lifestyle and health. In J. Watson & S. Platt (Eds.), *Researching health promotion* (pp. 54–78). London: Routledge Press.

Anheier, H. K., Gerhards, J., & Romo, F. P. (1995). Forms of capital and social structure in cultural fields: Examining Bourdieu's social topography. *American Journal of Sociology, 100*, 859–903.

Antonovsky, A. (1996). The salutogenic model as a theory to guide health promotion. *Health Promotion International, 11*, 11–18.

Archer, M. (1996). *Culture and agency: The place of culture in social theory.* Cambridge: Cambridge University Press.

Berkman, L. F., & Breslow, L. (1983). *Health and ways of living: The Alameda county study.* New York: Oxford University Press.

Berkman, L. F., & Kawachi, I. (2000). *Social epidemiology.* New York: Oxford University Press.

Blaxter, M. (1990). *Health and lifestyles.* London: Routledge Press.

Bourdieu, P. (1984). *Distinction: A social critique of the judgement of taste.* Cambridge, MA: Harvard University Press.

Bourdieu, P. (1986). The forms of capital. In J. G. Richardson (Ed.), *Handbook of theory and research for the sociology of education.* CT: Greenwood Press.

Bourdieu, P., & Passeron, J. C. (1990). *Reproduction in education, society and culture.* London: Sage Publications.

Cockerham, W. C. (2005). Health lifestyle theory and the convergence of agency and structure. *Journal of Health and Social Behaviour, 46,* 51–67.

Cockerham, W. C., Rütten, A., & Abel, T. (1997). Conceptualizing contemporary health lifestyles: Moving beyond Weber. *Sociological Quarterly, 38,* 321–342.

Davis, T. C., & Wolf, M. S. (2004). Health literacy: Implications for family medicine. *Family Medicine, 36,* 595–598.

Durkheim, E. (1997). *Suicide.* New York: Free Press.

Eysenbach, G., Powell, J., Kuss, O., & Sa, E. R. (2002). Empirical studies assessing the quality of health information for consumers on the World Wide Web. *Journal of the American Medical Association, 287,* 2691–2700.

Fowler, B. (1997). *Pierre Bourdieu and cultural theory: Critical investigations.* London: Sage Publications.

Freire, P. (1985). *The politics of education: Culture, power and liberation.* South Hadley, MA: Bergin & Garvey Publishers.

Frohlich, K. L., Corin, E., & Potvin, L. (2001). A theoretical proposal for the relationship between context and disease. *Sociology of Health and Illness, 23,* 776–797.

Frohlich, K. L., & Potvin, L. (1999). Collective lifestyles as the target for health promotion. *Canadian Journal of Public Health, 90,* 11–14.

Giddens, A. (1991). *Modernity and self-identity: Self and society in the late modern age.* Cambridge: Polity Press.

Hawe, P., & Shiell, A. (2000). Social capital and health promotion: A review. *Social Science and Medicine, 51,* 871–885.

Jenkins, R. (2002). *Pierre Bourdieu.* London: Routledge Press.

Kawachi, I. (2001). Social capital for health and human development. *Development, 44,* 31–35.

Kickbusch, I. (1986). Life-styles and health. *Social Science and Medicine, 22,* 117–124.

Kickbusch, I. (2001). Health literacy: Addressing the health and education divide. *Health Promotion International, 16,* 289–297.

Koenig, H. G., McCullough, M. E., & Larson, D. B. (2001). *Handbook of religion and health.* Oxford: Oxford University Press.

Krieger, N. (2003). Theories for social epidemiology in the twenty-first century: An ecosocial perspective. In R. Hofrichter (Ed.), *Health and social justice: Politics, ideology, and inequity in the distribution of disease.* San Francisco: Jossey-Bass.

Lane, J. F. (2000). *Pierre Bourdieu: A critical introduction.* London: Pluto Press.

Marmot, M., & Wilkinson, R. G. (1999). *Social determinants of health.* Oxford: Oxford University Press.

Martin, J. L. (2003). What is field theory? *American Journal of Sociology, 109,* 1–49.

Nutbeam, D. (2000). Health literacy as a public health goal: A challenge for contemporary health education and communication strategies into the 21st century. *Health Promotion International., 15,* 259–267.

Powell, L. H., Shahabi, L., & Thoresen, C. E. (2003). Religion and spirituality. *American Psychologist, 58*, 36–52.

Schwingel, M. (2003). *Pierre Bourdieu zur Einführung.* Hamburg: Junius-Verlag.

Siegrist, J., & Marmot, M. (2004). Health inequalities and the psychosocial environment—two scientific challenges. *Social Science and Medicine, 58*, 1463–1473.

Weber, M. (1978). *Economy and society: An outline of interpretive sociology.* Berkeley: University of California Press.

Williams, S. J. (1995). Theorising class, health and lifestyles: Can Bourdieu help us? *Sociology of Health & Illness, 17*, 577–604.

World Health Organization. (1986). Ottawa Charter for Health Promotion. *Health Promotion International, 1*, 405.

World Health Organization. (2000). *Glossar Gesundheitsförderung.* Hamburg: World Health Organization.

6

Understanding Differentiation of Health in Late Modernity by Use of Sociological Systems Theory[1]

JÜRGEN M. PELIKAN

1. Introduction: A Systems-Oriented Conceptual Framework for Defining, Observing, and Intervening in Human Health

To understand health as a social phenomenon in history, especially in modernity or in present late modernity, a refined conceptual framework of human health is needed. Such a framework, or even better, a model or a theory identifies defining and differentiating states, conditions and determinants of health as well as provides a foundation for practical applications to intervene into the production of health.

Within the context of this book, health is a concept as defined by the World Health Organization (WHO 1948)[2], on which the Ottawa Charter on Health Promotion (WHO 1986) also is based[3]. Therefore, the different states and multidimensionality of positive and ill health, the three-dimensionality of physical, mental and social

---

[1] This as any of the other chapters owes much to the intensive process of discussions between the authors of the different chapters of this book. My thinking concerning health in late modernity also has been influenced continuously by my colleagues at the Institute of Sociology and the LBISHM of the University of Vienna, especially Rudolf Forster, Karl Krajic, Christina Dietscher, Wolfgang Dür, Peter Nowak und Ursula Trummer. The text has profited considerably by discussions with and reading by Marina Fischer-Kowalski and professional editing by Andrea Neiman. Thanks also go to my assistants Katrin Uhlik and Simone Grandy and my secretary Brigitte Frotzler for different kinds of support in preparing this chapter.

[2] Health is a state of complete physical, mental and social well-being and not merely the absence of disease or infirmity. (WHO 1948)

[3] Health promotion is the process of enabling people to increase control over, and to improve, their health. To reach a state of complete physical, mental and social well-being, an individual or group must be able to identify and to realize aspirations, to satisfy needs, and to change or cope with the environment. Health is therefore, seen as a resource for everyday life, not the objective of living. Health is a positive concept emphasizing social and personal resources, as well as physical capacities. Therefore, health promotion is not just the responsibility of the health sector, but goes beyond healthy life-styles to well-being. (WHO 1986)

health, and the distinction of health as a subjective experience on the one hand, an objective resource or capacity on the other hand, should be, and is represented. It is in this chapter, that the concept of health shall be further explored and explained within the basic context of (sociological) systems theory.

Indeed, it is the purpose of this chapter to provide an understanding of the widening and differentiation of social processes relating to health in late modernity. This chapter introduces, employs, criticizes and develops the neo-classical (as compared to Talcott Parsons classical) systems theory of the German sociologists Niklas Luhmann (1927–1998), as it relates to health matters. This kind of universal social theory offers concepts that help to differentiate between traditional and modern society from a macro, meso and micro perspective, as well as allows describing specific features of present society in late modernity. Yet, sociological systems theory has been applied to analyses of health only marginally. Therefore, it will be necessary to further specify and develop some health related key concepts. This mainly holds true for a systemic understanding of human physical, mental and social positive and ill health. Based on a rather complex definition, employing Luhmann's not less complex conceptual framework for function systems, an analysis of health care and public health in modernity, and of health related services and health promotion in late modernity is offered. By that, the chapter focuses on the understanding *of* health in modernity by sociological systems theory. The other interesting perspective, how a better use of sociological systems theory *in* health care and public health could improve their effectiveness, is left for another publication. By its universal character, sociological systems theory is rather abstract and somewhat tedious to follow. So, probably is reading this chapter. Hopefully, the extra effort will be rewarded by some relevant insights into more adequately approaching and improving health in late modernity, insights to be gained best when using systems theory.

2. Health of Living Systems: A Quality Generated by Reproduction of the Living System in Its Environment

In systems theory the starting distinction for observing phenomena is the difference of **system** vs. its (relevant) **environment**. For a **living** system this implies that the system has to **reproduce** itself continuously or it will die as a system. The living system has to produce its distinct identity, specifically its boundaries, by itself, but within a relevant environment. To maintain itself, a living system has to relate to its environment, partly by fencing itself off from it, to stay distinct, and partly by using its resources, to reproduce itself. Therefore, problems of closure and openness need to be addressed within and by a living system. The concepts of autopoiesis and structural coupling, developed by Maturana and Varela (Maturana and Varela 1987), and introduced by Luhmann (Luhmann 1997; Luhmann 1995) into the sociological systems theory, provide one specific way to model these problems. To keep its specific identity in an environment, a living system has to be able to use the difference of system vs. environment within the operations of the system. In other words, observation of self must be distinguished from observation of non-self. Within this kind of framing, reproduction of a system at a certain point in time has to be understood partly as determined and influenced by the history and the characteristics of the system itself and partly by characteristics of the systems' relevant environment. That will have consequences not only for understanding the re-production of health attributed to a living system, but also for possibilities of intentionally influencing the natural or generic reproduction of the system by specific interventions. These starting assumptions may sound rather abstract as they stand now, but they will become much more concrete in the course of this chapter.

The result of ongoing or past reproduction of a living system can be judged as more or less successful, with respect to the variety of present and future options for the system, from the perspective of the system itself or from an external observer. As far as the present state of the system is concerned, two dimensions can be distinguished: the degree of positive (well-) or negative (mal-)**functioning** (or disablement), and the degree of positive (well-feeling) or negative (mal-feeling) **self-experiencing** of the system. Both can be combined to actual well-(or mal-) **being** of the system. With respect to the future of the system, the two most important dimensions are expected quantity, i.e. **longevity**, of survival (measured as life expectancy) and expected quality of future living, i.e. **quality of life**. Both dimensions sometimes are measured in combination by Disability Adjusted Life Years (DALY's). These two capacities are what we will be addressing as the living systems "**health**". Good health is defined to be a good capacity for survival and enjoyment of life. **Ill health** (illness, sickness and disease, impairment and disablement) means that a living system has a restricted capacity for survival and enjoyment of life. So health and illness mostly as unintended but more and more also as intended consequences of living are profoundly related to the very existence and reproduction of a living system. Using these two perspectives the system can observe, monitor and evaluate itself, or be observed, monitored and evaluated by others. But health and illness are rather broad and complex umbrella concepts, under which the actual and future existence, functioning and experiencing of living systems can be addressed. Later, when we discuss societal reactions to health and illness, we will have to look again at differing consequences of their specific aspects for societal attention, cultural formation and opportunities for intervention.

To describe the reproduction of a living system in more detail, it is necessary to distinguish between **structures** vs. **processes** of the system, separating the living system itself from the environment in which it lives. Structures can be understood as patterns of related elements; processes can be understood as patterns of related events or operations occurring in time. Using Weick's (Weick 1976; Weick 1985; Weick 1995) terminology, structures are described best as patterns of more strictly coupled elements as against processes as patterns of more loosely coupled events. Therefore structures usually frame or condition processes, but in time also structures can be changed or developed by processes. The behaviour of a living system is determined by its anatomy, but in time behaviour may develop anatomy in a certain direction, as could be observed impressively with Arnold Schwarzenegger, when he was a young man.

Following quality theory (Donabedian 1966; Donabedian 1990) or the European Foundation of Quality Management-model (EFQM 1999), structures and processes together can be understood as **enablers** for specific **outcomes** (or outputs) of the system, or for **effects** (or impacts) the system has on its environment. Usually outcomes and effects are understood as intended by specific actions of the system, whilst outputs and impacts just happen as a consequence of ongoing behavior of the system. Therefore, outcomes and effects are conceived as specific subsets of outputs and impacts. This kind of thinking has been developed for business organizations as a specific type of social systems first and later been adapted for non profit organizations (NPO's) as well, but it can be generalized for all kinds of systems, including living systems.

Like in quality philosophy, healthy as a specific criterion of quality cannot only be applied to outputs or outcomes, but to structures and processes of a system as well. This kind of thinking includes the assumption that healthy structures are a precondition for healthy processes, and both are preconditions for healthy outputs/ outcomes. From that also follows that health determines health, or health (in the past) is the best predictor for health (in the future). This statement formally is tautological, but it is also empirically true. For the health related qualification of structures and processes of a living system, a specific terminology was introduced by Aaron Antonovsky. Ongoing reproduction or living may result in more or less **salutogenic**, i.e. health producing, (Antonovsky 1979; Antonovsky 1996), or **pathogenic**, i.e. also illness producing, structures and processes, measured by their fulfillment of—or deviation from—normal or ideal types of appearance, or by their correlated effects on health or illness of the system in the future. The same kind of classification following the same kind of logic can be used for characteristics of relevant environments of living systems; they can also be classified as more or less salutogenic or pathogenic for the reproduction of specific living systems (cf. Figure 6.1). A similar distinction may be drawn between salutogenic **resources** and pathogenic **risk-factors**, and applied to characteristics of living systems as well as to characteristics of their relevant environments. Within the ecological discourse oriented at sustainability, the effects of the reproduction of a system on its environment are observed: The relevant distinction here is whether these effects of system reproduction are making this environment more or less salutogenic or pathogenic for the quantity and quality of survival of this or similar kinds of living systems in the future.

We still need to clarify the specific distinction between **health** and **illness** and what kind of relationship can be specified between the two concepts (Pelikan and Halbmayer 1999). Within our model of reproduction of a living system within an environment, both health and illness have to be seen as determinants as well as results of the ongoing reproduction or living of the system. Reproduction usually produces health, as a precondition for further survival, but eventually reproduction will also generate illness, as a precondition for (premature) death. In more concrete

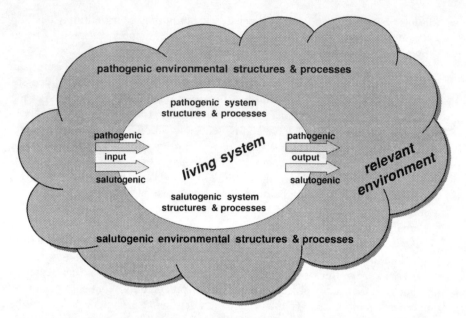

FIGURE 6.1. Schematic representation of salutogenic and pathogenic structures, processes, inputs and outputs relevant for a living system interacting with its relevant environment.

terms, we can speak of **positive** health as something that is enabling for (better) survival and 'fighting' against **negative** or ill health, or illness. With that distinction, we can define a formula for the relationship of positive and ill health to health: the amount of total health of a living system is its amount of positive health minus its amount of illness. (Of course it could be debated, if the relation should be regarded as additive, but this seems to be a simple and plausible assumption.) At the same time, one has to be aware of an important asymmetry between the two: positive health can exist without illness, but illness always needs a minimum of positive health to host it, so to speak. So, logically, it would be more correct to speak of illness "of" or "within" health, than of illness "and" health. (Metaphorically, we could understand the relationship of the two as one of host and parasite.) Therefore, it does not make much sense to treat (positive) health and illness as opposites, as some do. Only death and life form an either-or-relationship, and even here in case of dying, i.e. crossing in terms of Spencer Brown, there seems to be some zone of indifference, depending on the method of observation. In contrast, (positive) health and illness do co-exist with each other, at least for a broad section of the spectrum. Only lethal illness will eat up (positive) health totally, in time. So one should better treat (positive) health and illness as the extreme poles of a continuum of different mixtures of positive health and illness, with optimal positive health without any disease at one end, and minimal positive health with a maximum of disease at the other (cf. Figure 6.2).

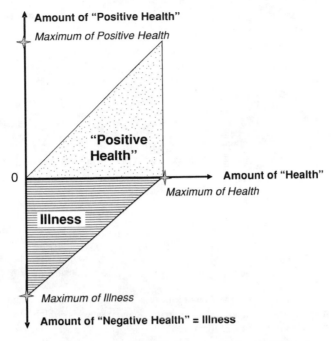

FIGURE 6.2. Schematic representation of positive and negative health jointly constituting a health continuum.

(Positive) health and illness do co-exist, but not independently from each other in time. Since, good positive health is a precondition to control and fight illness, and illness has the potential to reduce positive health in the future. So, positive health is endangered by illness and by accidents, but also by another kind of biological process, ageing. Aging, partly depending on the kind of living, will, to a certain extent, reduce or limit positive health, following the life-cycle of an organism.

There also is another important asymmetry concerning the appearance and extension, and by that also the perceptibility and definability of positive and negative health. Positive health usually is taken for granted as a normal, given, general, diffuse, unconscious, rather latent or virtual state of being. In contrast, ill health, especially acute ill health, is experienced as a deviant or aberrant, specific, manifest or actual state, or even as a dramatic event, which by experience of pain, discomfort and disablement forces attention and reactive action. Ill health makes a difference by interrupting and changing the quality of everyday life, often in a way not to be turned down. Ill health introduces a new specific quality of functioning and experiencing, while it is difficult to distinguish positive health as something specific and distinct from everyday survival, living, or living well. So we will not be surprised to find that societies and individuals have a much more elaborated code for perceiving and observing ill health, and react with priority to manifestations of ill health, while good health may remain relatively unnoticed. Looking at

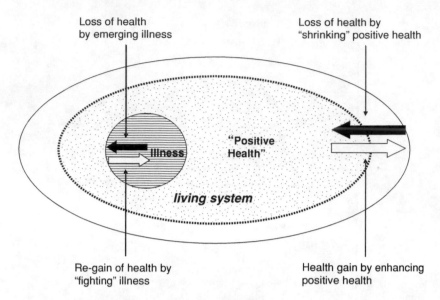

FIGURE 6.3. Schematic representation of illness as a parasite of positive health. A model by which 4 different kinds of health related outcomes and processes, which can be intervened separately or in combination, are identified.

positive and negative health as a continuum, ill health does vary between better marked extremes, namely absence of ill health and death, while positive health can vary from some minimal quantity of living up to some kind of ideal, optimal, maximum quantity of well-functioning and well-feeling. Notwithstanding these considerable differences in appearance and experience, both these relevant and valued qualities associated with living can be influenced and changed by focused human attention and directed interventions into the preconditions, structures, and processes, of living.

For practical reasons it is important to observe both positive health and illness independently (cf. Figure 6.3), and be aware that there are different specific determinants for positive health, mainly resources, and for illnesses, mainly risk-factors, and therefore health and illness can be influenced directly and independently, but by processes of interaction they will also have indirect effects on each other.

So positive health and ill health do not only vary independently to a certain degree, but in human society both can also be maintained and improved by four different and independent principal strategies (cf. Table 6.1). In more detail, these strategies are:

– reactive **treatment** of actual illness or impairment (by measures of specific cure and general care),
– prophylactic **prevention** of future illness and impairment (by controlling specific risk factors),

TABLE 6.1. Principal strategies to maintain and improve human health

Oriented at	Positive health	Ill health
Maintaining health	Protection of positive health	Prevention of ill health
Improving health	Development of positive health (including rehabilitation)	Treatment of ill health

– proactive **protection** of positive health (by controlling of functioning—no over-, under- or misuse—and by providing sufficient and adequate general resources, and by specific protective measures) and
– **development** of positive health (through specific training and exercise, including rehabilitation after impairments by illness and accidents).

The distinctions or boundaries of these four strategies are somewhat fuzzy, especially that between prevention and protection. Often to be most effective, the strategies better are applied in combination, e.g. treatment and protection, but also protection and prevention or treatment and development.

Taking into account that interventions can address the system and/or its environment, a more complicated picture arises (cf. Table 6.2). Depending upon the

TABLE 6.2. Principal strategies to maintain and improve health by influencing living systems & relevant environments

Oriented at	Positive health	Ill health	Positive health	Ill health
By influencing	System	System	Environment	Environment
Maintaining health	**Protection of positive health** by improving individual resource-management	**Prevention of ill health** by improving individual risk-management	**Protection of positive health** by developing infra-structures & incentives for resource-management	**Prevention of ill health** by developing less risky environments & incentives for risk-management
Specific intervention	*(Health education for positive health protecting lifestyles)*	*(Health education for ill health preventing lifestyles)*	*(Development of resourceful living conditions)*	*(Development of less risky living conditions)*
Improving health	**Development of positive health** by improving individual exercise & training	**Treatment of ill health** by cure & care for individuals	**Development of positive health** by investing in infra-structures & incentives for exercise & training	**Treatment of ill health** by investing in infra-structures & incentives for cure & care
Specific intervention	*(Health education for health promoting lifestyles)*	*(Self-/ lay-/ professional management of illness)*	*(Development of health promoting living conditions)*	*(Development of specific conditions for management of illness)*

strict or loose, structural or operative, coupling of system and relevant environments, the effectiveness and efficiency of these interventions will be different. It will be more direct and visible and therefore also more spectacular, to intervene in the actual pathogeneity of the system (and less so in the pathogeneity of its relevant environment) and less direct and visible to intervene in the salutogenicity of the system (and even less so in the salutogenicity of its relevant environments). But, interventions in environments can improve the health of many different living systems at the same time, and investments in the salutogenicity of a system can improve its resistance to many different potential illnesses within a long time span in the future. So any serious comparison of health related strategies of intervention or investment has to take into account factors of scale and time.

This conceptual model for the health of living systems, admittedly and already, bears a certain complexity, a complexity that cannot be reduced without risking a serious distortion of the reconstruction of the health reality. Nevertheless, the conceptual model will have to become even more complex, when we try to specify it for more specific phenomena of human health.

2.1. Human Health: Result of the Interplay Between Three Different Systems, Constituting the Human Individual

What is the **system** in question in the case of **human health**? The answer, of course, depends upon the perspective we choose. We are well advised to take a broad rather than too narrow a perspective. So we start with the human individual as the basic carrier of the quality called "health". Following sociological systems theory and respecting the WHO definition of health, we cannot describe the human individual as just one system. Rather, following a paradigm or model proposed by Luhmann (Luhmann 1990), and specified by Simon (Simon 1995), Pelikan & Halbmayer (Pelikan and Halbmayer 1999), Bauer et al. (Bauer et al. 2003, Bauer Davies and Pelikan 2006), we will have to understand the individual as the structural and operational coupling of three different kinds of systems. The three coupled autopoietic systems are: an organism or body, a mind or mental system (consciousness in Luhmann's terms) and a social status or a person (again in Luhmann's terminology) (cf. Figure 6.4).

Why three different systems? Because: organism, mind and person have to reproduce themselves by different basic operations, using different kinds of environments that cannot be reduced to one another. Organisms reproduce metabolically, minds with ongoing thoughts, and persons by communication, especially communication of decisions with other persons or collective social actors. Of course, there is no natural person or mind without a living organism as a material basis. Mind and person are better to be understood as evolving co-evolutionary on the basis of a living organism. But in an extreme case, a body can be kept alive without a functioning mind, and—socially—still be treated as a person. So for the three systems constituting the human individual, there is certain independence, represented by autopoiesis, and certain interdependence, represented by structural

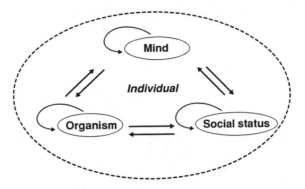

FIGURE 6.4. The individual as a structural coupling of three systems: organism, mind and social status.

and operative coupling. Interdependence also means circular causal influences of the organism on the mind and the person, but also the other way round from the person on mind and the organism. For living, or for purposes of reproduction, the three systems of the individual have to rely on and use each other: The body is needed to act out plans developed by the mind, which, in due time, could develop qualities of the body, and by that, might change experiences of the mind as well. For example, if the mind thinks, that a trained body is more attractive, he perhaps makes his body go for a run every day. The consequences of the trained body may be not only a better functioning body and more positive attention socially but a mind that feels more in control as well. For taking part in social communication, the mind (for selecting information and understanding messages) as well as the body (for perceiving and sending messages) is needed. The social status of a person is limited by the experiences of the mind and the actions of the body, but, over time, decisions of the mind and actions of the body can develop the social status of the person in the future. As far as social status is concerned, processes of individual performance and achievement and societal processes of ascription and access together determine the social position of an individual in every social system.

Within a lifetime, or in ontogenesis, the opportunities for development, the flexibilities for change and the general variety of the three systems are different: for the body they are more biologically limited, for the mind they are more flexible by use of symbolic learning, and are, at least in modern open societies, most open for variation of the social status of the individual. From that also follows that body and mind are more strictly coupled than the person is either to mind or to body. In human history there was much less biological evolution of the human body, compared to the cultural evolution of the human mind, and even less compared to the social evolution of possible social status of the person in society. There is much less possible variation between adult human beings for the amount of their physical strength, compared to their amount of knowledge or their wealth.

TABLE 6.3. The three systems and relevant
environments of the human individual

Dimensions/levels	System	Environments
physical	organism	nature
mental	mind	culture
social	person	society

All three types of systems are further differentiated within themselves, the organism into biological subsystems or organs, the mind into psychological subsystems, and the person by inclusion and participation in different types of social systems. In modernity the most relevant of these are the family, education, economy, law and politics.

What are the relevant **environments** for conditioning or influencing reproduction of organisms, minds and social persons? Here, we can only give a rather abstract answer: there is a bio-chemical-physical material environment relevant for the metabolism of the organism, a perceivable and meaningfully coded cultural environment for the psycho-cultural reproduction of the mind, and a socio-economic environment of society, as a hybrid of the material and the cultural, for the socio-economic reproduction of the person (cf. Table 6.3).

Again, no society (of a human population, material artifacts and social institutions) and no culture (symbolic language and other kinds of semantics) persists without a material or living substrate. And again, a co-evolutionary relationship of society and culture has to be assumed. As far as necessary conditions and causal influences are concerned, the material environment influences primarily the reproduction of the organism, the cultural environment primarily the reproduction of the mind and the socio-economic environment primarily the reproduction of the social status of the person.

What does that mean for human positive or ill **health**? We have to distinguish between three different kinds of positive and three different kinds of ill health, all in all between 6 dimensions and types of indicators for human health (cf. Table 6.4)

TABLE 6.4. Dimensions and indicators for positive and Ill health relating to the three systems of the human individual

Systems of the individual	Positive health	Ill health
Organism	Physical well-functioning and well-being (fitness & wellness)	Accidents & actual and chronic diseases
Mind	Mental well-functioning and well-feeling (fitness & wellness)	Mental disturbances & actual and chronic mental diseases
Person	Social inclusion in relevant societal sub-systems & participation in social resources (citizenship, formal education, work, family & social networks, wealth, prestige etc.)	Acute & chronic personal social deviances (illegality, analphabetism, unemployment, poverty, social isolation, being an outcast etc.)

TABLE 6.5. Salutogenic and pathogenic factors in the three types of relevant environments for human individuals or populations

Enviroments	Salutogenic	Pathgogenic
Nature	Basic metabolic contexts & resources (climate, air, water, food, light etc.)	Acute natural catastrophes & detrimental chronic conditions (e.g. pollution) & scarcety of necessary resources
Culture	Basic cultural orientations & values (like tolerance,	Anomia; ethnocentrism, fundamentalism
Society	Basic societal institutions & resources (peace, justice, wealth, social capital, trust, etc.)	Acute & chronic detrimental societal conditions (e.g. war, civil war, terror, instability, extreme inequality, extreme competition)

Correspondingly we can name salutogenic and pathogenic factors in the relevant environments for the health of organism, mind and person (cf. Table 6.5).

Taken together, we get a complex multi-factor model of natural or generic health development (Bauer, Davies, and Pelikan 2006) which specifies a complex etiology of health and illness and by that also allows for a variety of specific interventions to advance and promote health in a systematic and purposeful way. So this model also should be an adequate basis for reconstructing the social organization of dealing with health and illness within different types of society.

2.2. Summary

Within the framework of systems theory major differences are introduced to specify matters relating to human health. These differences mainly are system vs. environment; structure & process of systems vs. its output, outcome or impact; positive vs. ill health as an output of systems reproduction; salutogenic (infrastructures & resources) vs. pathogenic (risk factors) characteristics of systems & their environments; physical vs. mental vs. social positive & ill health of human individuals characterized by organism, mind and social status within relevant environments of nature, culture & society. Together and in combination these differences describe a complex health space with multiple opportunities for etiology of and social interventions in health and illness. As will be shown in the following analysis, societies differ in the way they use different parts of this health space to socially deal with health and illness. Clinical medicine and public health seem to be extremely differing approaches in dealing with health policy.

3. Health in Modernity

To adequately describe, analyze and understand specific practices of and discourses on health in late modernity[4] we have to bear in mind the broader context of the

---

[4] Late modernity (or liquid modernity) is a term for the concept that some present highly developed societies are continuing developments of modernity. A number of social theorists

meaning and processing of health in modernity[5]. Until now, a general conceptual framework for defining health, and strategies of health care, public health and health promotion has been developed. What still is missing is an adequate scheme for understanding (late) modernity. By modernity we mean the context of modern versus some kind of traditional society, and by late modernity, we mean the present developed phase of modernity. Some (e.g. Lyotard 1984) like to call this phase post-modernity or postmodern society, but we prefer following e.g. Giddens (1991) to speak of the **late modern society** and leave the term post-modern for a specific discourse of self-description within late modern society. To proceed with our health focusing endeavor, we do need a clear understanding of modern and late modern society. Sociological systems theory does help to clarify these concepts.

Using neo-classical sociological systems theory a la Luhmann, modern society can be described as a specific type of society, characterized by a specific mixture of types of social differentiation. Modern society primarily is differentiated functionally, and only secondarily by stratification and segmentation. Segmentation is denoting that similar social parts exist side by side; stratification is identifying different social parts ordered hierarchically. Whilst **functional differentiation** is defined by principally different, specialized social parts functioning autonomously side by side but inter-dependent by some kind of division of labor. Functional differentiation in this type of societal theory is seen as the basis of **individualization** and **globalization**, world-wide **urbanization**, and of what some would call a society of **organizations**. It is thus, functional differentiation of different societal sectors that is seen as the root of some of the most discussed tendencies, forces or dynamics of the present global or world society. It is useful that sociological systems theory—as a principally universal kind of theory—has something to say on these important phenomena. But, in our context the dominant question is, what follows from functional differentiation for the analysis of health in modernity? To answer this, we first will need a better understanding of the meaning of functional differentiation.

Functional differentiation assumes that in modern society there exists at the macro level specific function systems, at the meso level specific types of organizations, and at the micro level specific social roles have evolved. These social systems or arrangements do fulfill important functions for the whole of society, as well as

---

(Beck 1992, Giddens 1991, Lash 1990) critique the idea that some contemporary societies have moved into a new stage of development or postmodernity. On technological and social changes since the 1960s, the concept of "late modernity" proposes that contemporary societies are a clear continuation of modern institutional transitions and cultural developments. (Wikipedia 2006, http://en.wikipedia.org/wiki/Late_modernity)

[5] Modern can mean all of post-medieval European history, in the context of dividing history into three large epochs: Antiquity or Ancient history, the Middle ages, and Modern. It is also applied specifically to the period beginning somewhere between 1870 and 1910, through the present, and even more specifically to the 1910–1960 period. (Wikipedia 2006, http://en.wikipedia.org/wiki/Late_modernity)

solve problems and/or offer solutions, achievements, performances necessary for the functioning of other function systems, as well as for organizations and individuals. In contrast to Parsons (1951) theory of social systems, Luhmann notes that the number and the specific kinds of function systems cannot be deducted or do not follow logically from theory. To Luhmann, there remains as an empirical question what sort of and how many function systems have evolved in societal evolution so far. There is consensus within the community of sociological systems theory that at least economy, politics, law, religion, education, art, science, mass media and family can be observed or reconstructed as distinct function systems in modernity. But there is disagreement and discussion within the scientific community, if e.g. social work or nursing should be treated as fully developed and differentiated function systems

Function systems are defined as a specific type of social system as compared to interaction systems, organizations or society at large. But as social systems they have in common to be communication systems, i.e. their elements are communicative events in time. A communicative event is seen as a sequence of three selections: the selection of *information*—for a *message* by alter, which is selected for *understanding* as a message, and not just perceived as information by ego (in terms of the framing of double contingency, shared by Luhmann with Parsons). Further, function systems, as with any other social systems, are understood as autopoietic systems, meaning they have to produce the communicative events, they consist of or operate with by themselves—meaning, in a self-referential, operationally closed manner. To make this improbable communicative processes happen, function systems in general do use binary codes (like true/false in science) for their closure or demarcation of boundaries, and programs (like theories and methods in the case of science) for their openness to relate to relevant environments. Some do also make use of symbolic generalized media (truth in the case of science) to make acceptance of their specific communications more probable and have developed symbiotic mechanisms (like perception in the case of science) as a specific form of relating to the human body of the persons involved. Some have developed specific reflection theories (like theory of science for the function system of science) to reflect and try to control their self-steering in societal evolution. These concepts are the instruments that sociological systems theory offers for analyzing the social processing of health in modern society. Within this paradigm of modern society, regarding to matters of health, at least two types of questions arise. First, is there at least one or are there even more distinct and specific function systems, specialized in processing problems of human health in modern society? And second, what is the meaning of health as a reference in other function systems, fulfilling primarily their different specific functions, e.g. meaning, in science, are there developing specific sciences related to health? For the first type of question, an answer has been given by systems theory, but an answer upon which critical thought and improvement can occur. Concerning the second question, there is not much of a tradition in system theory to follow this line of thinking, but of course, this then provides an opportunity to begin.

3.1. Medicine or Care of Ill Health As a Specific Function System in Modern Society

Luhmann has not written a specific monograph, as he has done on the major function systems, on health care or medicine, but he has published three papers related to health in modern society (Luhmann 1983a; Luhmann 1983b; Luhmann 1990). In these papers he assumes that there has evolved a specific function system dealing with health in modern society which he interchangeably called "treatment of disease", "treatment of ill persons" or "medicine", not carefully distinguishing between the three terms. Using the general characteristics, he had developed for analyzing function systems, he characterized, what here will be called the "function system for care of ill health", with ill/healthy as the binary code and diagnostic methods and therapies as programs. He also assumed that, in contrast to other function systems, health care has not developed a specific generalized symbolic means of communication, a symbiotic mechanism nor a complex theory of reflection. But, as he describes doctor/patient as the specific role relationship for including persons in this function system, he mentions the hospital and medical practice as a specific type of organization of this function system.

Luhmann's system theoretical analysis of health care has not been taken up much in sociological or medical sociological literature, with two major exceptions: **Bauch** (Bauch 1996; Bauch 2000a; Bauch 2000b) and of **Pelikan** et al. (Pelikan and Halbmayer 1999; Bauer et al. 2003; Bauer, Davies, and Pelikan 2006; Forster, Krajic, and Pelikan 2004). Bauch in most respects follows Luhmann's analysis, but he criticizes him for not taking into account newer health related developments and therefore proposes a much wider binary code; that of hindering vs. promoting health or even life.

Pelikan et al. follows Luhmann in a number of respects, but furthers his application of some of the general concepts related to the specific case of health. Besides that, they try to make use of the WHO definition of health and the developments it stimulated, especially as it relates to the Ottawa Charter of Health Promotion.

For analysing a function system, the definition of the binary code is decisive, because it marks its identity and boundaries. Luhmann here opted for illness vs. health or ill vs. healthy. Illness or ill is stated as the value of connectivity (to start interventions) and health or healthy the value of reflection (to stop interventions). This specification can be questioned, theoretically as well as empirically. Empirically, it can be argued that for a long time health care, or medicine, did not actually use positive health as a reflection value, but limited itself to the management of illness. Medicine has been criticized, by medical sociology, social medicine and other critics (e.g. Illich) for limiting itself to a medicine of repair. In its actual practice, as compared to its self-description, medicine uses "absence of disease" as a value of reflection or stopping rule, and "presence of disease" as a value of connectivity or an entrée billet to its area of responsibility. Therefore, at least for a certain period in modern history, the binary code of health care or medicine can be described more adequately as presence vs. absence of illness (broader) or of disease (more narrow). Theoretically, two arguments can be made. First, from Luhmann's own judgment that medicine has not yet developed a proper reflection theory follows that health as the value for reflection has not been properly specified for any practical use. Second, accepting the argument developed earlier in this chapter that only death and life are logically proper opposites, but positive health and illness do co-exist besides each other over a broad spectrum, and do follow different salutogenic and pathogenic etiologies, and furthermore, can be influenced by different types of interventions; it does not make sense to combine them in one code, but rather to specify two different codes, and relate these to physical health, specifically. These could be presence vs. absence of *physical* illness (disease) for ill *physical* health. For positive *physical* health, a somewhat more complicated construction has to be proposed: suboptimal vs. optimal *physical* positive health. An observed deficit in actual positive *physical* health, as the value of connectivity, would allow for starting some kind of intervention, and a theoretically or empirically defined criterion of optimal positive *physical* health—as the value of reflection—would serve to define some kind of stop rule for ending the intervention. Of course, the two binary codes can be combined in more complex programs of medical practice, like in surgery, where anaestiseologists are responsible for the patients' positive health, so that surgeons can concentrate on dealing with the pathogenic aspects. It can and will be argued that the success of modern medicine, historically, is related first to its focusing on care of ill *physical* health or disease. But, in late modernity it can be observed that medicine is more and more following the code related to influencing positive *physical* health as well. Therefore, medicine and cure of disease are no longer identical, but are becoming differentiated. So, medicine more and more grows into the shoes of "health care", in the proper and broader meaning of the term.

·But, before we follow this line of reasoning further, we must first analyze modern medicine or the system of **care of ill physical health**. Referring to the code of presence vs. absence of physical ill health successful diagnostic and therapeutic **programs** have been developed, jointly by clinical medical science and clinical medical practice, based upon natural science knowledge of the functioning of the human organism. But what about a specific **medium** of communication and a specific symbiotic **mechanism** for the function system of curing physical ill health? Luhmann, and Bauch (who follows Luhmanns argumentation) do claim, that there is none. This claim seems to be problematic. It can be argued that the science-based system of medical terminology for differential diagnostics, even codified internationally in the ICD[6], and for the related system of therapies, defined in

---

[6] International Classification of Diseases (ICD):ICD-10 was endorsed by the Forty-third World Health Assembly in May 1990 and came into use in WHO Member States as from 1994. The classification is the latest in a series which has its origins in the 1850s. The first edition, known as the International List of Causes of Death, was adopted by the International Statistical Institute in 1893. WHO took over the responsibility for the ICD at its creation in 1948 when the Sixth Revision, which included causes of morbidity for the first time, was published. The ICD has become the international standard diagnostic classification for all general epidemiological and many health management purposes. These include the analysis of the general health situation of population groups and monitoring of the incidence and

medical textbooks, handbooks, journals and reviews, constitute such a medium. This medium fulfills the criterion of enhancing the probability of acceptance of specific actions, i.e. a specific diagnosis followed by a specific, often highly risky, but still accepted therapy. This medium is not only, but mostly, used in the function system of cure of ill health between doctor and patient (and relatives), and between the different professional providers of cure and care. It is also used in other function systems, like medical research, medical education, and increasingly in economics, politics, mass media and by lay people in everyday life.

There also can be observed at least three different kinds of practices which fulfill the criteria of symbiotic mechanisms, i.e. linking the medium to the human body, like physical force (by police and military) does for the medium of power and governance in politics. In the case of curing ill health, these are the more sophisticated and successful diagnostic and therapeutic interventions for the human body—i.e. pharmacy, surgery, radiology (and laboratory medicine). The fact that there is no well-developed **theory of reflection** for the function system of curing ill health, as Luhmann and Bauch state, and as empirically seems to be true, also can be explained using our assumptions. "Absence of..." as the simple value of reflection within the binary code, together with the presence of a practically extremely successful medium of communication and symbiotic mechanisms, speak for themselves, and do not need any specific theoretical reflective legitimating, in contrast to the function systems of politics or education or of public health and health promotion, for that matter.

The specific semantic medium "medical terminology" of the function system for care of ill health allows for a **first** kind of **structural coupling** of the clinical core of this system with two other function systems, **scientific research** and **education**. This coupling is also partly institutionalized in the multi-functional organizational unit medical clinic and the professional role of the (chief) doctor of the clinic. Both institutional arrangements do combine ill health care, scientific research and educative training functions, because the clinical core of all three is in need of the presence of real patients to interact with. A **second** kind of structural coupling with the function system of **economy** is made possible by the main symbiotic mechanisms of ill health cure—pharmacy, surgery, radiology, laboratory medicine—which all allow for and do rely on technical procedures, apparatus and artifacts, which can be produced and distributed as individual goods by the industrial market economy with profit for a partly guaranteed and continuously expanding world market. This kind of structural coupling of the techno-medical complex does guarantee financing of planned continuous scientific and technical

---

prevalence of diseases and other health problems in relation to other variables such as the characteristics and circumstances of the individuals affected. It is used to classify diseases and other health problems recorded on many types of health and vital records including death certificates and hospital records. In addition to enabling the storage and retrieval of diagnostic information for clinical and epidemiological purposes, these records also provide the basis for the compilation of national mortality and morbidity statistics by WHO Member States. (WHO 2006, http://www.who.int/classifications/icd/en/)

innovation of medical cure and care for ill health, and it assists in making it an industry of growth. A **third** kind of structural coupling can be found with the function system of **politics** or with the state. The strength of this coupling does vary considerably with the kind of political system in which it is developed and promoted. It was and in very few cases still is stronger for real socialist state societies, and it is rather stronger for European welfare states than for more neo-liberal market societies like the USA. Since ill health care always is dealing with the integrity of the body, and more and more of life itself, the practice of ill health care is legally regulated by politics in all modern societies. As examples of stem-cell therapy show, there is a growing demand for legal regulations of new possibilities for interventions that result from scientific progress. But, politics has not always limited itself to regulate who is allowed to do what kind of repair of the body without sanctions. In various political systems, to some extent, politics also has taken responsibility for organizing and providing supply and financing of ill health care. This willingness to take so much political responsibility for health care is rational, since care of ill health is not only a private good in great demand by anybody who is seriously ill, but it is in the interest of society and its members to treat health as a public good. Systems theory oriented analysis of ill health in modern societies shows that not only a thorough understanding of the functioning of the specialized system of caring for ill health is necessary, but also of the relations of this system to other function systems in its relevant societal environment. Sociological systems theory offers a paradigm and concepts that are fit for both types of analysis

3.2. Public Health in Modern Society

The modern state was and is, as far as health is concerned, not only engaged in regulating, organizing and financing care and cure of ill health for individuals but the modern state (as cities and imperia before) was and is also dealing with issues of public health. How is the social place of public health to be understood in modern functionally differentiated society? Has there evolved a distinct and specific function system for public health besides the function system for care of the individual ill health? Or, has public health rather emerged as a set of several specific sub-systems in different function systems like science, education and politics? And, if the latter, what keeps public health together as an identical unity across the function systems which host specific aspects of it? If, first, we look for specific **social structures**, especially for a dominant and specific type of institutionalization, what can we find? Schools, departments, institutes, projects of public health as far as organizational units are concerned. Journals, books, web-sites and other forms of publications as specific public media relating to public health; interactive communication events or processes like conferences, meetings, seminars, workshops for public health. And, specific legislation, budgets, programs and policies address issues of public health in politics. So, we do find quite a number of structures and events with public health as a "sign on the door" (cf. McQueen, chap.). But, do they together form a distinct function system? The answer has to be, no! All institutional arrangements we find can be assigned either to the function systems of science, education, politics or mass media, as subdivisions, with specific reference to public health. Second, is there a distinct **role-relationship** for inclusion of individuals and other actors, specific for public health? Also, not! Rather, the usual role relationships of the function systems in question are used: teacher/student, researcher/user of knowledge, politician (civil servant)/citizen, author/reader. But it could be argued that a new more abstract kind of role relationship is emerging, that of public health expert/client. This relationship does not lead to a new specific function system, but is realized within the context of other already existing function systems, like the public media or politics. Finally, can we define a specific societal **function** for public health? Yes! This function could be defined as "prevention of physical (mental and social) ill health and protection of physical (mental and social) positive health of specific populations by developing less pathogenic environments (and stimulating less pathogenic behaviours)". So, it focuses upon two principle strategies of maintaining and improving health (cf. Table 6.11). This function is not fulfilled by the emergence of a distinct and specific function system of its own, but taken over mainly by politics, relying upon and using solutions, achievements, performances of science, law, and—to a lesser degree—education and the mass media.

Even if we cannot find distinct social structures, but rather sub-structures in other function systems, there has to have evolved a specific **semantic** for public health, if only to allow for public health specific sub-divisions in other function systems to emerge. The binary **code** for public health could be formulated as presence vs. absence of pathogenic (risk) factors in environments (including infrastructures and behaviours of populations). The respective public health **programs**, making this code operational by specifying theories and methods for monitoring of and for interventions into environmental and population risk factors are very heterogeneous due to the many dimensions involved in the development of healthy environments. For changing unhealthy behaviours of individuals and populations, these programs go in the direction of "health education" and media campaigns. There is also the development of a specific domain of public health knowledge. But this does neither rest on sufficient evidence and consensus, nor does it invite improbable behaviour to happen to a degree that would fulfil the criteria of a generalized symbolic **medium** of communication, like it seems to be the case for clinical medicine. Without that kind of specific medium, there is also no specific **symbiotic mechanism** to be expected relating to individual bodies. (As far as health education is considered, the mechanism involved is not related directly to the human body, but to the human mind, and therefore has to use the general means of social communication, and rely on individual perception and learning). Also, a well developed **theory of reflection** can not be expected, since the value of reflection for public health is absence of pathogenic risk factors, which makes an extended theory of reflection neither possible nor necessary.

So, what keeps public health together as a social unity? Semantically, a shared code and a variety of shared programs, which facilitates accumulating shared specific knowledge. Concerning its social structure, a first answer could be, public health is a **social movement**, with the aim of assuring and improving the health of populations. Until now, this movementhas to a certain extent been successful in initiating and using research, law, education and mass media communication for planning, implementing and legitimising specific public health policies and programs. A second social arrangement is the **coupling** of the different function systems involved, by individuals holding positions in organisations relating to different systems at a time (multi-position holders), or are mobile (as go betweens) between the systems in their career over time. And a third, intensive **referencing** (e.g. in decision making) of the involved systems on each other, e.g. public health education, public health mass media communication and public health politics on public health research.

But, why has public health not been as successful as (clinical) medicine or the other social movements for health in modernity, which has developed into a specific and remarkably growing function system? If we take the amount of research money and publications, or the number of professionals involved, or money spent on interventions as empirical indicators for success, the answer becomes even more interesting if we accept that clinical medicine has made and is making a smaller contribution to fighting (infectious) disease and increasing life expectancy than measures of public health (Lalonde 1974; McKeown 1976). For a fair answer to this question, we have to discuss the principal differences between the two fields or disciplines in more detail.

Clinical medicine is oriented to treat actual, manifest and severe ill health of single individuals, whereas public health is oriented at avoiding future, possible ill health of abstract populations. (E.g. the medical diagnosis of lung cancer is inviting for a number of possible therapeutic reactions, which will have a probable effect on survival and quality of life of the individual concerned, whereas public health best can assure smoke-free areas which will decrease the probable risk of developing lung cancer in the future.) So medicine is addressing problems of life or death of present individuals, whereas public health is promising to prevent future health problems in abstract populations. Medicine can focus its interventions on individual organisms, whereas public health has to intervene into social living conditions, life-styles and environments of populations, i.e. into the functioning of society itself. So the focus of medicine is more narrow and stable in principle, whereas social living conditions or environments of individual humans are not only much wider, but historically constantly changing over time. For effective diagnosis and therapy, medicine has to rely upon natural and clinical sciences only, whereas public health also needs the less developed psychological and social sciences for effective interventions in human behaviour and society. For medical interventions partly standardized technical solutions are possible, which lead to marketable individual goods, products and services for big populations, forming the basis for an ill health industry of continuous growth, in contrast public health can only partly be addressed with technical solutions; public health depends heavily upon social interventions in social conditions, processes and behaviours. Individuals can be isolated for a specific time span for treatment in specific organizations of a distinct health care function system, which is specialized in the caring of ill bodies, and is dominated by the medical profession. For public health to be effective, it has to intervene continuously on the daily functioning of *all* organizations in *all* function systems, especially into the economy, and in personal behaviour of *all* individuals. Therefore, the practice of public health is basically political or educational, i.e. trying to influence collective binding decisions for better health from the local to the global level. For technically intervening into human bodies, medicine as a profession has a monopoly and license, whereas the profession of public health just has a specific expert knowledge and an expert status in political, educational and mass media debates. Even for that, public health always has to rely on clinical medical diagnosis, aetiology and epidemiological research to prove that a certain characteristic of an environment or a human behaviour is pathogenic or a risk for health.

4. Health in Late Modernity

In the last few decades there can be observed considerable changes in societal processing of health. They possibly can and should be understood as manifestations of more general processes and changes in modernity. Following the understanding of modernity as the "project of modernity" (Habermas), modernity has to have a beginning and an end, and can be structured internally into historical phases. There is much speculation about the end of modernity, or even of history (Fukuyama), resulting in propositions of various post-isms: post-modernity (Lyotard), post-industrialism (Bell), post-work-society (Offe) to experience-society (Schulze), post-class-society to life-style society, post-capitalist to information- or knowledge-society, market-economy to market-society.

But how can we construct something like "late" modernity in a theoretical systems perspective? For sociological systems theory, the socially constitutive characteristic of modernity is the primacy of functional differentiation. And functional differentiation is associated with the rise and growth of various types of function system specific organizations, world-wide globalization of function systems and their organizations, and individualization of single human beings, integrated into society not by lifelong embedding to one multifunctional social unit, but by principal inclusion and actual decided participation in many different function-systems by taking complementary roles. All this also applies to late modernity. These distinctive modern tendencies rather are extended to regions and populations where they have not yet been present, and are intensified, where they already have existed in the past. That particularly holds true for economic transformations from agrarian to industrial to service-based modes of production, with corresponding processes of urbanization.

The period since the late 1980's is characterized by a specific intensification of globalization of information, capital, goods, services and workforce, so dramatically experienced by the people that the term and phenomenon is thought to be new, and not a process that has been occurring for many centuries already. This intensification is partly the result of political processes, the break-down of real socialism, the end of the cold war and of bipolar political situation. But it is also supported by new or better technologies of transport, of (tele-) communication and data-processing, by digitalization and miniaturization of products, like computers, telephones etc. and the creation of the world wide web. Some of the health related changes associated with late modernity are: basic transformations of clinical medicine or care of ill health, a growing fitness and wellness industry, the rise of health promotion as an avant-garde of a new public health, to name only three. These changes, if judged as dramatic and sustainable enough, could justify a new kind of diagnosis for late modern society, the diagnosis of "health society" (cf. Kickbusch chap in this book) instead of a "medicalized society" for old modernity, competing with or substituting older diagnoses like "risk society" (Beck) or "information society" or "knowledge society" (Willke). Before we will look at health, we better get some basic understanding of some more trends and events that make late modernity different to "old" modernity.

As far as the dimension of **social differentiation** is concerned, the primary functional differentiation in the centres of a developing world society is intensified by further differentiation and specialization of function systems, already present in modern, and to a greater extent in more traditional nation states in the peripheries. By intensification and expansion of functional differentiation, further processes of **globalization** are made possible, since it is function systems and their organizations that can be globalized across national borders. Therefore, organization dominated society is also progressing. The same holds also true for **individualization**. Individualization is the result of the dissolution and reduction of functions of productive and reproductive households and communities for integrating individuals into society. Due to this phenomenon, these individuals are set free to be actively included and participate in different function systems, to take complementary roles in the specific organizations of these, as consumers, citizens and patients.

4.1. Health Care for Individuals in Late Modernity

At least four different, partly complementary developments can be observed:

1. We can observe a **transformation of clinical medicine** from a profession predominantly curing ill health to a profession more and more of also improving positive physical health and quality of life for individuals. With that, medicine still remains oriented at the individual body and technical interventions into the structure and technical controls of processes of the functioning of the human body. What is expanded are the causes for interventions from diseases or the consequences of accidents to natural or socially defined deficiencies of optimal functioning or appearance of the body. So medicine develops around its disease-oriented core and expands to the periphery to address other aspects of human biology. Such areas include, reproductive medicine of fertility, fertility control and birth, via substitutive gendered medicines of aging (promising eternal youth) to palliative medicine of death; From changing unwanted primary sexual organs or orientations (medicine of sexual change), unwanted physical looks (beauty medicine), unsatisfying fitness

(sports medicine) and wellness, unwanted personal or social behaviours (e.g. over- or under-activity) (medicine of life-style drugs) to unsatisfying genetic structures, "new" medicine offers a lot more than just the curing of diseases.

This expansion of medicine can be interpreted as medicalization of life and living, i.e. making medicine responsible for diagnosing, treating and controlling a whole basket of life problems besides illness and disease. Medicalization partly can be based on pathologization, i.e. a pathogenic definition of or perspective on deficits or problems of the body, the psyche or social behaviour. Medicine's expansion into services of improving quality of health and life is another factor of rising costs for health care which necessitates new and better definitions of the boundaries of public or solidarity funded systems of care of (ill) health. (Inclusion of viagra in health care schemes is a good example for that kind of challenge.)

2. **Economizing of care of ill health**: The demand for care of ill health is rising continuously for many reasons. Some of the most pronounced are: changing demographics of global population (aging and individualisation of households), epidemiology of morbidity (shift from infectious epidemics to greater burden of chronic diseases, accidents and new epidemics) as well increased opportunities for medical interventions (scientific and technological innovations and progress), leading to rising (public and/or private) expenditures for care of ill health. This has stimulated different measures for cost containment for cure and care. Some strategies are applied to make clinical care more effective and efficient by standardization like Evidence Based Medicine (EBM), Evidence Based Nursing (EBN), disease-management and different forms of quality management. Some introduce financial incentives like Diagnose Related Groups (DRGs) or co-payments for users to decrease the amount of usage of (higher quality levels of) care and duration of care. Another tendency is introducing market elements into national health service systems (e.g. purchaser-provider split in the UK) or more organisation into market systems (e.g. Health Maintenance Organisations (HMOs) in the USA). So the whole ill health care sector is not only continuously increasing its share of GNP, but it is in permanent reform as well. Partly care of ill health is changing from a professional service to an industry of ill health care, with medical doctors loosing influence on the system, and managers and shareholders gaining it. From (chronic) patients a more active and responsible, self-caring and co-productive role is expected, with more health-literacy to navigate and use the system effectively and efficiently. From the perspective of (poor) patients these economizing strategies also result in reducing inclusion in the system of care for ill health, and may lead to new forms of exclusion of specific groups of vulnerable individuals.

3. There seems to happen a further **differentiation of care for ill health** into three different and separate, but institutionally partly overlapping systems for physical ill health (medical care), mental ill health (psychotherapy) and social ill health (social work), which principally can be described by using Luhmann's paradigm and concepts for function systems (cf. Table 6.6). Similarly there emerge, partly parallel, partly overlapping, function systems for developing **positive** physical **health** (sports and fitness training), positive mental health (meditation and wellness training) and social positive health (different forms of legal, economic and

TABLE 6.6. Different function systems for physical, mental and ill health, in late modernity

Name	Care of ill physical health	Psychotherapy	Social work
Semantics			
Code	Presence/absence of physical ill health	Presence/absence of mental ill health	Presence/absence of social ill health (social problems)
Programs	Modern clinical bio-medicine; complementary "old" medicines	Different (scientific) schools of psychotherapy, alternative/ complementary	Different schools of social work
Medium of communication	Codified knowledge of clinical medicine, specific diagnosis justifying specific therapies	Codified knowledge of psychotherapies and clinical psychology, specific mental diagnoses justifying specific communication therapies	Codified knowledge of social work, sociology, social psychology, specific diagnoses of social problems justifying specific social interventions; Partly money
Symbiotic mechanism	Diagnostic & therapeutic techniques to intervene the individual body (invasive diagnostics, radiology, surgery (transplantation), pharmaceutics, stem cells, genetic manipulation etc.)	Techniques of therapeutic communication	None
Theory of reflection	Since the reflection value is the absence of a physical deviance/ disturbance, not much of a reflection theory is necessary or possible. But: Evidence-Based-Medicine!	Since the reflection value is the absence of a mental deviance/disturbance, not much of a reflection theory is necessary or possible.	Since the reflection value is the absence of a social deviance/ disturbance, not much of a reflection theory is necessary or possible.
Structure			
Function	Treatment of (severe) ill health	Treatment of (severe) mental ill health	Treatment of (severe) social problems
Role relationship	Doctor (health professional)/patient	Psychotherapist/ mental patient	Social worker/client
Organization	Hospital, ambulance, medical practice, nursing home etc.	Psychiatric hospital, psychotherapeutic practice/ambulance	Different organisations of social work

TABLE 6.7. Different function systems for physical, mental and social positive health, in late modernity

Name		Physical fitness	Mental wellness	Social wealth
Semantics	**Code**	Suboptimal/optimal individual positive physical health	Suboptimal/optimal individual positive mental health	Suboptimal/optimal individual social wealth
	Programs	Of sports, gymnastics, physical fitness, rehabilitation	Health psychology. Health education, alternative/complementary spiritual cultural systems	Different forms of consultancy, coaching
	Medium of communication	Codified knowledge of biology, sports sciences etc. allowing for diagnosis of potentials and justifying specific treatment interventions	Codified knowledge of psychology, religious and spiritual systems	Codified knowledge for diagnosis of potentials & solutions of improving different aspects of social status
	Symbiotic mechanism	Techniques of training the body, anabolica etc.	Techniques of meditation	None
	Theory of reflection	Since the reflection value is optimal physical health, a reflection theory at least has to specify meaning and benchmarks for that.	Since the reflection value is optimal mental health, a reflection theory at least has to specify meaning and benchmarks for that.	Since the reflection value is optimal social health, a reflection theory at least has to specify meaning and benchmarks for that.
Structure	**Function**	Specific support for development of individual physical fitness and wellness	Specific support for development of individual positive mental fitness and wellness	Specific support for development of individual social resources (economic & social capital)
	Role relationship	Physical trainer (physiotherapist)/client	Mental trainer/client	Consultant/client
	Organization	Different organisations, (e.g. fitness-, sports-, rehabilitation-centers) providing infrastructures & services	Different organisations offering services for developing mental wellness	Different organisations of consultancy

social consultancy and coaching). These also principally can be described by using Luhmann's paradigm and concepts for function systems (cf. Table 6.7).

4. The growing importance of **health** as a point of secondary reference **in other function systems**, health related policies in politics, health related products, services and organizational policies in economics, health related information in the mass media, health related contents in education. On the part of individuals this corresponds to a growing amount of health related information seeking, communication and decision making in everyday life.

4.2. New Public Health in Late Modernity

For the transformation of old public health into some kind of new public health, the health promotion movement as an avant-garde within and outside public health was decisive. By definition, the notion of public health does relate to the health of populations on the one hand, and to collective actors responsible for or in a position to assure and improve health of these populations on the other. Historically, these collective actors responsible for population health have been cities in the first place, and later, with the rise of modernity, primarily (nation) states. In late modernity the types and number of collective actors in a position to care for public health policies have increased. After World War II a new global or world level has been created by the formation of the United Nations, with World Health Organization (WHO) as a specific subunit responsible for matters of health. Later, also other supranational agencies, like the World Bank, Food and Agriculture Organisation of the United Nations (FAO) and others have engaged themselves in public health programs on a global level. So a global public health discourse has been established, supported by "Global Health Reports", "The Millennium Goals for Global Health", and specific inter- or trans-national projects. WHO also engages in international initiatives to systematically improve public health on a national (WHO 1999) or regional level such as the Healthy Cities or Healthy Regions Initiatives. It is through these types of programs that the importance of the collective local level for public health has been strengthened. But following the Ottawa Charter (WHO 1986), WHO did not only focus on region based communities and their (local) capacity to work in public health, but also underlined the relevance of sector or function specific organisations, like schools, universities, prisons, workplaces and hospitals that also affect public health. It is because of this that the WHO started specific health promotion oriented networks for these types of organisations. Only health promotion in the workplace could build upon a public health tradition, dating back to at least to the 19th century, whilst other settings more or less have been identified as new partners for health.

In summary, **one** typically late modern ongoing tendency is the diversification and spread of responsible collective actors or settings. A **second** is the widening of attention from mainly fighting pathogenic risk-factors to also building up and strengthening salutogenic resources for health. A **third** is a widening of attention to include besides factors in the environment affecting health also behavioural factors such as individual styles of life and work. This tendency is a reaction to ongoing individualism and to changing risks and choices. To influence population behaviour as methods health education and specific public campaigns relating to specific health issues are being used. A **fourth** change also reacted on changes in epidemiology towards more chronic diseases and also increasing individual-isation of a better educated and more autonomous populations, by transforming more expert dominated solutions into more participatory kinds of problem solving, stressing enablement, empowerment and generating of health literacy for dealing with health problems, to allow users for shared decision making, co-production in cure and care and self-responsible healthy life-styles.

By these transformations, public health began to adapt itself to more general fundamental changes, like increasing globalization, individualization, "society of organisations" and to relative affluence. But the challenge of health promotion and a new public health only partially has been taken up and integrated into (this) old concept of public health. Partly, a separate process of institutionalization of health promotion, outside of the realm of public health, has been explored, with more or less success.

But compared to individual oriented types of societal processing of health, which have become more differentiated and varied, more evidence-based and standardized as well, with an even greater growth in late modernity, population oriented public health approaches have not gained adequate momentum. Population health and even more so a health promoting environment intrinsically has the quality of a public good and has to be promoted through joint and participatory political decision making, action and investment. In forming a global society with strong neo-liberal tendencies, with weakening of national welfare states, especially, coupled with the strengthening of market economy, towards some kind of "market society", the chances for investments into and growth of new or old public health are not particular promising.

5. Closing Comments

Sociological systems theory has been used to reconstruct the societal processing of health in modernity and late modernity. Its paradigm and concepts allow for a systematic analysis of specific characteristic, structures and semantics of modern societies and their consequences for social processing of health. The systems theory was also helpful in describing and interpreting actual tendencies and characteristics of late modern society, triggering new forms of health related phenomena. Varying emergent practices have been analyzed, specifically addressing the medical care of ill health and public health, with health promotion as an avant-garde or reform movement of a New Public Health paradigm. However, sociological system theory has been used more to reconstruct the different emerging systems *of* health related practices in (late) modernity, than to introduce the use of sociological systems theory *in* these health advancement practices. The latter could be seen as a potential to improve the effectiveness and efficiency of the professional practice of public health and health promotion, but this has to be left for another publication.

References

Antonovsky, A. (1979). *Health, stress and coping. New perspectives on mental and physical well-being.* San Francisco/CA: Jossey-Bass.

Antonovsky, A. (1996). The salutogenic model as a theory to guide health promotion. *Health Promotion International, 11,* 11–18.

Bauch, J. (1996). *Gesundheit als sozialer Code. Von der Vergesellschaftung des Gesundheitswesens zur Medikalisierung der Gesellschaft.* Weinheim, München: Juventa.

Bauch, J. (2000a). *Medizinsoziologie.* München, Wien: Oldenburg.

Bauch, J. (2000b). Selbst- und Fremdbeschreibung des Gesundheitswesens. In Henk de Berg and Johannes Schmidt (Eds.), *Rezeption und Reflexion. Zur Resonanz der Systemtheorie Niklas Luhmanns außerhalb der Soziologie.* Frankfurt/ Main: Suhrkamp.

Bauer, G., Davies, J. K., & Pelikan, J. M. (2006). The EUPHID Health Development Model for the Classification of Public Health Indicators. *Health Promotion International,* Advance Access published online January 9, 2006.

Bauer, G., Davies, J. K., Pelikan, J. M., et al. (2003). Advancing a theoretical model for public health and health promotion indicator development. Proposal from the EUPHID consortium. *European Journal of Public Health, 13*(Supplement), 107–113.

Beck, U. (1992). *Risk society: Towards a new modernity.* London: Sage Publication.

Donabedian, A. (1966). Evaluating the quality of medical care. *The Milbank Memorial Fund Quarterly, XLIV*(3), 166–206.

Donabedian, A. (1990). The seven pillars of quality. *Archives of Pathology and Laboratory Medicine, 114,* 1115–1118.

EFQM. (2000). *Vision and mission.* 22-7-1999.

Forster, R., Krajic, K., & Pelikan, J. M. (2004). Reformbedarf und Reformwirklichkeit des österreichischen Gesundheitswesens. In Oskar Meggeneder (Ed.), *Reformbedarf und Reformwirklichkeit des österreichischen Gesundheitswesens. Was sagt die Wissenschaft dazu?* Frankfurt/Main: Mabuse Verlag.

Giddens, A. (1991). *The consequences of modernity.* Cambridge: Polity Press.

Lalonde, M. (1974). *A new perspective on the health of Canadians.* Ottawa: Information Canada.

Lash, S. (1990). *The sociology of postmodernism.* London: Routledge.

Luhmann, N. (1983a). Anspruchsinflation im Krankheitssystem. Eine Stellungnahme aus gesellschaftstheoretischer Sicht. In Philipp Herder-Dorneich and Alexander Schuller (Eds.), *Die Anspruchsspirale: Schicksal oder Systemdefekt? 3. Köllner Kolloquium.* Stuttgart: Kohlhammer.

Luhmann, N. (1983b). Medizin und Gesellschaftstheorie. *Medizin Mensch Gesellschaft, 8,* 168–175.

Luhmann, N. (1990). Der medizinische Code. In Niklas Luhmann (Ed.), *Soziologische Aufklärung 5. Konstruktivistische Perspektiven.* Opladen: Westdeutscher Verlag.

Luhmann, N. (1995). *Social systems.* Stanford, CA: Stanford University Press.

Luhmann, N. (1997). *Die Gesellschaft der Gesellschaft.* Frankfurt am Main: Suhrkamp.

Lyotard, J. (1984). *The postmodern condition: A report on knowledge.* Manchester: Manchester University Press.

Maturana, H. R., & Varela, F. J. (1987). *Der Baum der Erkenntnis.* Bern: Scherz.

McKeown, T. (1976). *The role of medicine: Dream, mirage and nemesis.* London: Nuffield Provincial Hospitals Trust.

Parsons, T. (1951). *The social system.* New York: The Free Press of Glencoe.

Pelikan, J. M., & Halbmayer, E. (1999). Gesundheitswissenschaftliche Grundlagen zur Strategie des Gesundheitsfördernden Krankenhauses. In Jürgen M. Pelikan and Stephan Wolff (Eds.), *Das gesundheitsfördernde Krankenhaus. Konzepte und Beispiele zur Entwicklung einer lernenden Organisation.* Weinheim, München: Juventa.

Simon, F. B. (1995). *Die andere Seite der Gesundheit. Ansätze einer systemischen Krankheits- und Therapietheorie.* Heidelberg: Carl-Auer-Systeme.

Weick, K. E. (1976). Educational organizations as loosely coupled systems. *Administrative Science Quarterly, 21*, 1–19.

Weick, K. E. (1985). *Der Prozeß des Organisierens*. Frankfurt a.M.

Weick, K. E. (1995). *Sensemaking in organizations*. Thousand Oaks, CA: Sage.

World Health Organization. (1948). *Constitution.*

World Health Organization. (1986). *Ottawa Charter for Health Promotion (WHO/HPR/ HEP/95.1.)*. Genf: WHO.

World Health Organization. (1999). *Health for all: One common goal*. Genf, Schweiz: WHO.

World Health Organization. (2006). *International Classification of Diseases (ICD)*. http://www.who.int/classifications/icd/en/

7
Managing Uncertainty Through Participation

LOUISE POTVIN

1. Introduction

Participation enjoys a very special status in health promotion discourse. Conceptualised both as a process and a valued outcome, it is often viewed as a defining feature and a key principle of health promotion (Robertson & Minkler, 1994; Rootman, Goodstadt, Potvin & Springett, 2001). Taking advantage of an undisputable position as a cardinal value, the role of participation has rarely been critically examined in relation to health promotion practice and its contribution to public health. The questions regarding the role of participation and how, in practice, practitioners can facilitate and support its emergence, have not been given satisfactory answers. Answers to these crucial questions can only result from a theoretical understanding of what participation entails in terms of action in the social situations of health promotion interventions. Theorizing on the role of participation in health promotion and on the social processes at play when it occurs is a prerequisite to reframing participation as a professional practice rather than as an ideology (see Pelikan, Chapter 6), and to develop appropriate procedures that can foster the conditions for effective participation.

Using social theory, this chapter seeks to shed a fresh light on the notion of participation. Firstly, identifying some of the reasons why the world in which we live is increasingly uncontrollable by scientific means (Giddens, 1990, 1994), this chapter will argue for the necessity of public health to develop a practice of participation as a strategy to manage the uncertainty associated with reflexivity, a characteristic of our contemporary society (see Balbo, Chapter 8). Secondly, expanding upon Callon's Actors Network Theory we will elaborate a theoretical conception of participation as a process by which groups of heterogeneous actors negotiate their role with regards to a social situation; in so doing these actors actively explore the possible worlds that can be collectively pursued.

2. Public Health and Reflexive Modernity

Public health is the combination of science, practical skills, and values directed to the maintenance and improvement of the health of all the people. It is a set of efforts organised by society to protect, promote, and restore the people's health through collective and social action (Last, 1998, p. 6).

Like many authors who attempted to define public health, Last clearly associates public health with the modernist perspective of advancing the human condition through rationality and science to inform public choices and population management (MacKian, Elliott, Busby, et al., 2003). An exemplary endeavour of *The Enlightenment*, public health rests on the underlying assumption that the association of science and the State through expert knowledge and bureaucracy will yield to a world where disease and death, conceived as failures of nature, are no longer part of the human experience (Fassin, 1996). "Suffering, healing, and dying, which are essentially transitive activities that culture taught each man, are now claimed by technocracy as new areas of policy-making and are treated as malfunctions from which populations ought to be institutionally relieved" (Illich, 1975, p. 132). Although public health can certainly claim to have fulfilled a great deal of this command, its action also generated novel sanitary challenges. Using Giddens and Beck's critic of modernity, this section explores how these challenges come about.

Over the past 150 years through various interventions, programs and initiatives, public health as an institution has significantly contributed to improving the health of populations and in so doing, built a convincing case for the do-ability of health (see Kickbusch, Chapter 9). In fact, many of the public health achievements, such as the global eradication of smallpox or the reversal of the cardiovascular mortality trend in the 1970's, are truly spectacular. In health however, as in many other applied sciences, the modernist utopia of creating an orderly world through the application of scientific knowledge has been achieved often at the cost of creating new risks or adverse outcomes. The new realities engineered through scientific and technological progress are also associated with unexpected and undesirable outcomes (Beck, 1992, 2000; Giddens, 1994). Global pollution is the more obvious example of such unintended consequences.

In the health sector, the whole area of work on epidemiological transition shows how public health progress in longevity and disease prevention constantly lead the way to new sanitary challenges that were previously unforeseeable (Frenk, Bobadilla, Stern, et al., 1994). Like the previous transition periods that marked public health history (see Potvin & McQueen, Chapter 2), the third revolution of public health faces many new challenges that result from the successful efforts to control infectious diseases and to prevent chronic diseases; this in turn, limits the generalization of people's capacity to produce health equally throughout entire populations (see Abel, Chapter 5). The most frequently cited challenges are often associated with people's social conditions, such as: the increasing health disparities between those at the top of the social hierarchy and those at the bottom; the resurgence of infectious diseases, such as tuberculosis, in low income populations; the emergence of new epidemics due to changes in lifestyle (e.g. heart disease, obesity, diabetes) or outbreaks due to new viruses (e.g. HIV, SARS); the dramatic decrease in life expectancy in Sub-Saharan Africa and Eastern Europe; the population backlash against universal vaccination programs, and many others.

For many present-day sociologists and social critics, a major task of contemporary social theory is to explain this partial failure of science and rationality exemplified by instances where unintended consequences of scientific progress are identified after their negative impact is starting to be felt. For Beck, Giddens and Lash (1994), the reflexivity that inherently accompanies the development of knowledge is an essential ingredient for explaining why knowledge and scientific discoveries do not translate into more control over, and predictability of, nature and society.

According to many social theorists, reflexivity is a defining feature of modernity. For Giddens, reflexivity is one of the dynamic forces that lead to the transformation of institutions and that constantly impede our capacity to render our world more predictable. While self-reflection and a capacity to analyse one's own place in the world has been a feature of all societies (Beck, 1994; Giddens, 1994), reflexive modernity highlights a different dimension and a different role of knowledge in the transformation of societies.

The reflexivity that comes with modernity[1], together with unavoidable unintended consequences associated with technological developments (Beck, 1992), are the main reasons "why has the generalizing of sweet reason not produced a world subject to our prediction and control" (Giddens, 1990, p. 151). For Giddens, reflexivity primarily relates to the social practices involved in attempts to exercise control over aspects of our world, and how such practices continuously transform, and are transformed, by the knowledge they generate The fact that knowledge about the world is a part of the world blurs the relationship between knowing subjects and the objects of knowledge. Thus, knowledge gained about the world through science is constantly being reintroduced in society, participating to the latter's increasing complexity (see McQueen, Chapter 4). "The reflexivity of modern social life consists in the fact that social practices are constantly examined and re-formed in light of incoming information about those very practices, thus constitutively altering their character" (Giddens, 1990, p. 38).

Reflexivity implies that the relationships of social actors with institutions and other social structures are being transformed by scientific knowledge reintroduced into the social world via the media, the increased access to education and information, and through professional practice. In other words, the increasing level of knowledge about the functioning of society available to all social actors, contributes to altering their practice; the very object of that knowledge results in a pervasive gap in scientific knowledge and the objects of that knowledge. Through this double hermeneutic[2], the objects of expert knowledge are thus continuously transformed by it, creating a world in continuous transformation that can never be completely predictable. Consequently, the accumulation of knowledge about

---

[1] In the rest of this chapter we will adopt the term reflexive modernity (Lash, 1999) to label the contemporary version of modernity experienced in western societies (Beck, 1994).

[2] The first order of hermeneutic is that of the scientist interpreting the world. The second order is that of interpreting the effect of producing knowledge about the world has on the world and on the knowing process.

the social world and the gain in transparency associated with this accumulation, does not necessarily convert into a greater control over social development and evolution (Giddens, 1990, p. 16).

Another feature of reflexive modernity is the growing capacity of social actors to distance themselves from the influence of the social structure. In reflexive modernity, agency is progressively freed from structure (Lash, 1994) through increased individualization. This is the process by which individuals increasingly become the main decision makers on the matters of their life; the choices and chances that influence their lifestyles are less determined by the tradition or by social structures. "Individualization therefore means that the standard biography becomes a chosen biography, a do-it-yourself biography" (Beck, 1994, p. 15)[3]. An absolute prerequisite however for the fabrication of such a "reflexive biography" is access to information not only in terms of its availability but more importantly, in terms of the actor's capacity to interpret it and integrates its meaning (see Abel, Chapter 5).

As a consequence of the growing unpredictability of our social world and of the freeing of agency from the structure associated with reflexive modernity, the orientation of social changes in predictable directions through professional practice rooted in expert knowledge cannot be totally achieved. Instead of a clear and linear causal chain of events that link interventions to social changes, the implementation and unfolding of interventions in the real life is better represented as an open trajectory, at every point in time, a variety of scenarios could be, and effectively are, elaborated and selected. Furthermore, the range and content of those possible scenarios are incrementally unpredictable as time passes and contingent upon their context[4]. The future is always open and social actors can always radically modify a given course of action. Thus, when it comes to transforming social structures, the impact of interventions based on expert knowledge and technology can only be anticipated as plausible scenarios containing also a large dose of uncertainties[5].

As an institution characterized by a set of goals, a knowledge base and practices (see Last's definition above) public health should be largely concerned with reflexive modernity. Public health is about using scientific knowledge for transforming the world to increase people's longevity and decrease the burden of disease. The very act of assigning a public health meaning to a human experience is changing the reality of this experience, thus rendering somewhat less accurate the very knowledge that contributed to assigning this experience a meaning relevant to

---

[3] A significant dimension of this do-ability of one's own biography is the do-ability of one's own health (see Kickbush, Chapter 9).

[4] McQueen's chapter in this book discusses how contextualism, together with complexity and reflexivity, challenge the ability for health promotion to develop sound theoretical bases.

[5] One major difference between Giddens' and Beck's conceptions of late modernity lies in the generalisation of this conclusion to the natural world (Lash, 1994). Whereas Beck's *Risk Society* clearly extends the notion of reflexivity to humanity's attempts to rationally exploit and control nature, Giddens' reflexivity seems to be limited to social innovations. This discrepancy in their thinking is only tangentially related to the argument developed here since it is generally accepted that public health programs and interventions include important social components.

public health. An example of public health power to change the meaning of social realities is the labelling by public health of the current tendency for an increasing proportion of North American people to carry excess weight, as an obesity epidemic. This label actually conveys to these overweight people the message that they have a health problem instead of, or in addition to, one of body image. In so doing, it is changing the course of the phenomenon itself: people will not react the same way to health concerns as they do to aesthetic or moral concerns. As a result, public health is always confronting a reality that is being transformed by the knowledge it produces and by its practice to transform the reality. Thus, in public health as in many other techno-scientific endeavours, more knowledge does not necessarily translate into more predictability and control. It often means increasing complexity and uncertainty about the impact of action through unintended consequences and reflexivity.

To continue to be a relevant institution in reflexive modernity[6], public health must develop strategies and practices to manage this uncertainty. One such strategy lay in the confrontation of a multiplicity of perspectives about the situation and in the active exploration of a maximum of the plausible scenarios that are made possible, and are developing, in the course of action. Adding information, even contradictory, is a way of exploring such plausible scenarios (Callon, Lascoumes & Barthe, 2001). We will later argue that the management of uncertainty resulting from the reflexivity of social practices necessitates that the perspectives being considered and confronted include those of the broadest range of relevant actors. However, in order to properly examine how participation conceived as the confrontation of heterogeneous perspectives contributes to the management of uncertainty, one should first develop a theoretical understanding of the social actions and interactions that take place in situations of participation. And while health promotion is leading the way in advocating that public health practice include active participation, such a theoretically informed understanding is still lacking.

3. Programs as Public Health Practice

Practices of public health are broad and diverse and as illustrated in Last's definitions, they are essentially action-oriented. Most activities performed in the name of public health are concerned with the justification, design, implementation, or evaluation of actions that involve deliberate interventions to alter one or several processes that are thought to be harmful to the health of individuals or populations or promote and sustain healthy actions (Green & Kreuter, 1999). Public health interventions may take a variety of forms, however, three types dominate public health practice: public policy that regulates social actors' practice through sanctions and norms (e.g.: tobacco regulations; car seat belt laws, safety norms); the

---

[6] We mean by this public health capacity to influence the orientation of society in a way that is compatible with its goal of improving the health of the population.

development and maintenance of public infrastructures for people to use more or less freely (e.g. clean water, sanitation, bike paths); and programs in the sense of resources and knowledge to achieve specific goals (e.g. vaccination, diabetes prevention, community development). Although the question of participation is relevant to all of these forms, this discussion will mainly focus on programs.

Even if the term program is widely used in relation to public health interventions, attempts at defining its exact meaning and delineating its conceptual frontiers are scarce (Potvin, 2004). It is generally accepted that public health programs are composed of resources assembled to create and maintain activities and services designed and implemented to pursue specific objectives in response to a problematic situation that affects a target population in a specific context (Potvin, Haddad, & Frohlich, 2001). Using a spatial metaphor (MacKian, Elliot, Busby, et al., 2003), programs can also be characterized as social spaces: they involve network relationships between various social actors drawn together around a common interest; the aim being to create new meanings and/or relationships between actors relevant to the program's objectives. For example, a school-based smoking prevention program would endeavour to change the meaning of tobacco smoking for adolescents, assigning it a negative value, rather than an accepted and cool one. With respect to the space metaphor, those relationships and their content can be mapped to illustrate the general form of those networks, the relative distances between actors involved, as well as the content of these interactions. Also included in the task of modelling a program, is the establishment of a set of criteria that allows for the identification of those relationships that are considered within or outside of the program space.

3.1. Top-Down and Bottom-Up Public Health Programs

From the point of view of participation, the expressions "top down" and "bottom up" have often been used to contrast two ideal-types of programs.[7] In their ideal-type form, top down programs are oriented by a rigid vision of the changes to operate and what constitutes valid intermediary steps and end-points. This vision is primarily informed by scientific knowledge and often programs are conceived as empirical and real world tests of scientific knowledge (Nutbeam, Smith, & Catford, 1990). Their rationality is founded on the mastery of relevant technical and instrumental procedures. The legitimization of power lies in the recognised expertise of those actors who are imposing a scientifically informed vision on the other program's actors; the latter are being objectified to the extent that their own objectives and projects are doomed irrelevant for the program. These programs are planned as a series of steps, and their implementation aims at producing a chain of pre-determined events, as prescribed by expert scientific knowledge (Scheirer, 1994). Even if difficulties in following the set course of actions are encountered, a

---

[7] The Weberian concept of ideal-type refers to a bundle of proprieties that would define an ideal instantiation of an object but that may be not be found all at once empirically.

great deal of efforts is usually deployed to fit the implementation conditions with those experimented during the program development phase (Nutbeam, Smith, & Catford, 1990).

In terms of social space, program planners use their expert knowledge and power to identify the set of relevant actors and to assign each group of actors a specific role in the sequence of events and activities that form a program. Relationships between the actors follow a hierarchical structure. This means that experts, from the top of the hierarchy, control the principal nexus of decisions. At the bottom of the pyramid, program beneficiaries are objectified, in the sense that they constitute the object the program aims to change and the relationships that they entertain with each other are not usually considered to rest within the program space. Finally, the content of the transactions between program actors is constrained by the actors' role, the program's objectives and the logic model. The landscape of such program space is static and orderly. It can be easily bounded in time and space by a set of criteria that are manipulated by program designers, implemented by program staff, and experienced by the program's beneficiaries[8].

In health promotion and disease prevention, many community trials were designed by academic researchers in order to test specific hypotheses. The Minnesota Heart Health (Salonen, Kottke, Jacobs, et al., 1986), the Pawtuckett Heart Health (Lefebvre, Lasater, Carleton, et al., 1987), and the COMMIT trial (COMMIT Research Group, 1991), to name just a few, are examples of top down programs. Although these programs did provide room for implementation variations following differences in contexts, they constitute attempts to use scientific knowledge about health and its determinants to design and implement activities and services aimed at correcting problematic situations with little input from other sources. In these instances, the rationality rests essentially in the correspondence between the scientific knowledge about the problematic situation and its determinants, on the one hand, and the technical solutions that were fabricated and encapsulated within the programs, on the other hand.

At the other end of the spectrum, there exist programs that are much less rigidly organised, almost to the point that they might appear as being improvised. In their ideal forms, bottom up programs are dynamic social spaces in which various groups of actors negotiate and coordinate their actions to develop a common vision and implement the activities that may lead to the realisation of this common vision. Scientific knowledge is one among several types of knowledge mobilized to structure and inform such a social space. The vision and objectives of bottom-up programs result from the confrontation of expert objective epidemiological and other types of diagnosis with the subjective knowledge of the local conditions and with values as formulated by concerned actors. This means indeed that the development of vision and objectives in these programs follows a more organic process, iterative and context specific.

---

[8] These three categories of actors are mostly useful in top down type of programs. The flatter the relationships between program actors, the more likely the distinctions between these categories will be blurred.

These programs often have as a starting point a loose menu of activities that are more or less framed and reframed by program staff and local actors in a permanent negotiation process. Indeed, identifying the relevant actors and trying to engage with them often constitute the core of the initial activities (Bisset, Cargo, Delormier, et al., 2004). One property of the negotiation process that enhances the dynamic evolution of a program is its capacity to be responsive to the ever-changing conditions of the broader environment (Potvin, Cargo, McComber, et al., 2003). The minimally formalised initial conditions that characterize bottom up programs, lead to a variety of developments, some mostly unpredictable at the start of the enterprise (Potvin & Chabot, 2002). Some programs fade away shortly after being launched and others burgeon into projects and programs that have a strong history of renewing themselves.

This form of program represents an innovative practice in public health, marking a rupture with more traditional top down programs, and this is for two reasons. Firstly, because such programs take advantage of horizontal relationships between all categories of actors, complex systems are produced whose initial conditions cannot be controlled by experts, whose evolution cannot be planned in advance, and whose outcomes are mostly unpredictable. Even if health professionals could manipulate the formative stages of a program, they cannot diminish the impact of the existing relationships between the local actors who engage with the program, thus helping to shape the functioning of the program (Potvin & Chabot, 2002). Secondly, because numerous actors in such programs are identified as spokespersons for various relevant organisations or social groups, and because actors' participation can rarely be imposed, the program structure is more akin to that of a network, reaching out beyond the immediate circle of participants and target groups. Indeed one of the strengths of this public health practice is to be responsive to changes in environmental conditions through its capacity to engage with newly identified relevant actors (Potvin, Cargo, McComber, et al., 2003).

There is little doubt that the bottom up form of public health programs is chiefly identified with health promotion on the one hand, (Potvin, Gendron, Bilodeau et al., 2005; Potvin & Chabot, 2002), and would be widely perceived as being more favourable to participation on the other hand (Green et al., 1995) however participation is defined. Even if participation has been introduced in health care systems since the 1960's (White, 2000), its enshrinement as a key value and principle of health promotion (Rootman et al., 2001; Robertson & Minkler, 1994) has sealed its generalized and sustainable association with public health and health promotion. Although numerous essays on public participation are being published in the health promotion literature, there is a lack of critical analysis about participation in general and on the favourable conditions for its emergence, how it can be nurtured and how it affects programs (Zakus & Lysack, 1998)[9].

---

[9] One notable exception is a recent paper by Contandriopoulos (2004) in which the author uses Bourdieu's concepts of symbolic struggle and objectivation to analyze public participation in health care decision making.

3.2. *The Uncritical Public Health Rhetoric of Participation*

One striking feature of the literature on participation in relation to public health and health promotion is the abundance of expressions that are used interchangeably. The term participation is most often linked to a broad, non-specific, category of people: consumers, citizens, community, the public or lay participants (White, 2000). These categories refer to people that are outside of the health system in contrast to those who are inside, i.e. the public health experts, administrators, practitioners, and researchers[10].

In terms of top-down type programs, people from inside the health system, (i.e. the professional experts recognised as such through a series of institutional rules), are those in control of the program space and those from outside the system are the beneficiaries of program activities or services. It is the beneficiaries' objectified problems that the program is designed to solve. Feedback loops from those beneficiaries towards experts are scarce and rarely effective in modifying experts' practice. Conversely, in bottom up programs, the roles and relationships within the program space do not follow the inside/outside distinction. Diverse forms of knowledge are actively sought and valued to enrich and broaden program's perspective on issues of interest. Thus, for the remainder of the chapter participation will be used as a generic term to encompass: those practices that involve collaborative relationships in the form of exchanges of opinion, knowledge or other resources between various groups of actors concerned by, and willing to, devote time and resources to issues of relevance to health in order to participate in decision making regarding priorities, planning, implementation or evaluation of public health programs.

The health literature provides three broad frameworks for thinking about participation. The first one analyses participation in terms of a quantifiable characteristic, in the continuity of Arnstein's work (1969), whose eight-step ladder of citizen participation provides a rating of the degree of control exercised by citizens upon the program. One recent version of this work uses the concept of ownership to describe this sense of control over program features by various groups of actors involved in a program (Cargo et al., 2003; Green & Mercer, 2001). The second type focuses upon the program's features in which program beneficiaries are involved. Rifkin, Muller, & Bichmann (1988) designed a measurement instrument that identifies participation in five aspects of the program: leadership; needs identification; organisation; resource mobilization; and management. The work of Green et al. (1995) that resulted in an evaluation grid to assess the level of participation in health promotion is a synthesis of these two

---

[10] In reflexive modernity where specialized knowledge is widely available and where individuals are lifelong learners, this distinction between experts from inside the health systems and lay people of all sorts (consumer, patients citizens and so on) is increasingly blurred (see Balbo, this book, and Callon, Lascoume & Barthe, 2001). This state of affair renders even more relevant a conceptualisation of participation that transcends this distinction between expert and lay people.

types of framework. Finally, a third type highlights the ideological dimension of participation. Fournier and Potvin (1995) argue that underlining the promotion of participation are three potentially conflicting values, utilitarianism, democracy, and empowerment. These, in turn result in three forms of participation. Program efficiency is enhanced through utilitarian participation. Representation of beneficiary's diversity is increased through a democratic form. Finally people's control over the conditions of their health is improved though empowering participation[11].

Although such empirical descriptions of the quantity, program features, and values associated with participation are essential components for a comprehensive understanding of participation, they remain unsatisfactory. First, they all implicitly or explicitly reiterate the inside/outside of the health system distinction, making participation an asymmetrical process where health experts are allowing outsiders to have a voice in health matters. Lastly, none of these frameworks provide an analysis of the social processes at play when participation is implemented in health programs. In response to the lament that "as a specific technique, community participation is not well understood" (Zakus & Lysack, 1998, p. 3), the next section proposes a theoretical model of the social process at play in situations of participation. This model is based on the sociology of translation, a social theory that seeks to explain the dynamics of network expansion.

4. Actor Network Theory and Participation

The work of Michel Callon in the field of science and technology studies provides the basis for our conceptualisation of participation in health programs. For the past 25 years, Callon has conducted systematic observational studies on the sociology of knowledge development. He followed groups of researchers in their daily work, including their interactions and collaborative transactions with lay people, as they pursued their research objectives. His sociology of translation renamed, Actor Network Theory, offers a theoretical model for the social process leading to technical innovations. The analogy of innovation is relevant for health promotion programs in the sense that such programs constitute either a local adaptation of programs tried elsewhere or locally designed actions to address local issues. In both cases, programs are innovative set of actions in their local context. Therefore, the analytical categories developed in the course of Callon's work are relevant for the analysis of the collaborative process that develops between groups of actors in health promotion programs.

---

[11] This chapter does not address the issue of empowerment, even if for many commentators in health promotion the notions of empowerment and participation are often used together. We agree that a critical appraisal of the notion of empowerment is as important as that of participation, but we think that each notion should be examined for its own sake before they could be linked into a coherent theoretical framework.

In the next sections we will further develop the idea that programs are socio-technical networks that expand through translation processes and then examine how participation is a special case of such programs.

4.1. Programs as Socio Technical Networks

Callon's research program is an attempt to elaborate a theoretical framework for analysing the elaboration of scientific knowledge and applied technology. For Callon (1986, 1989a, 1989b), all scientific propositions are embedded within a network of actors, both human and non-human. Scientific facts are not revealed by nature to a passive scientific observer. Scientific propositions need to be elaborated through systems of action that include previous knowledge and work done by other scientists experimental, and/or measurement apparatus that form the know-how (or embodied knowledge) of a group of scientists, testing by other groups using a variety of other apparatus and techniques, and the utilisation into new technologies (Latour, 1991). For Callon, all of the knowledge, apparatus, technical skills, actions, and humans involved in this process form a socio-technical network (1989a). Furthermore, all of these specific entities (knowledge, apparatus, etc. . .) mobilized in any given socio-technical network can be conceptualised as "mouthpieces" for the broader categories of actors they represent (Akrich, Callon, & Latour, 1988b). It is only through the analysis of its position in a socio technical network that the meaning of any scientific proposition can be fully assessed (Callon, 1999).

The concept of socio-technical network can also be applied to health programs when understood as systems of action. Indeed, health promotion programs are composed of objectives, resources, knowledge, experts, lay people, staff members, and contextual elements all forming a composite of human and non-human actors. In any instantiation of a program, each of these categories of elements is actually represented by a few specific entities. The particular health experts, words used for defining the objectives, persons who are targeted by the program and so on, are all potential mouthpieces for the broader categories to which they belong. These actors, their actions and the social space they create form a socio-technical network. So the concept of socio-technical network used to analyse knowledge in the making can also be expanded to analyse the life of programs.

Another area of relevance of Callon's work to health promotion programs is the relationship between knowledge and action. One important distinction resulting from the social studies of science is the distinction between "science as made" and "science in the making" (Callon & Latour, 1991; Latour, 1989). Science as made is composed of the numerous scientific facts that are produced in laboratories and disseminated in the public domain as powerful and almost irrefutable assertions about the state of the world, once they had been validated within the realm of the scientific activity (e.g.: smoking tobacco increases the risk of lung cancer; regular practice of physical activity increases longevity). When they reach the public domain, scientific facts are essentially purified of the controversies and debates that surrounded them when they were being elaborated[12]. Science in the making is an account of the translation that transformed observations into scientific facts through a negotiation process between relevant human and non human actors. To become a scientific fact an observation needs to be integrated into a socio-technical network and this integration follows a translation process.

Knowledge results from a negotiation process between heterogeneous actors whose viewpoints and perspectives are not necessarily compatible a priori (Callon, 1999). For new knowledge to emerge there has to be a negotiation process made of transformations and trade offs. Propositions have to be modified: each contender taking into account his or her opponents' perspectives, and provide arguments that cannot be rejected. Knowledge is negotiated to the extent that it results from mutual concessions by emerging groups that attempt to agree while assessing the relative validity of their own arguments (Callon & Latour, 1991).

Not unlike science in the making, the practice of health promotion programs also involves translation, negotiation, transformations and compromises. Various bodies of knowledge have to negotiate their role in the construction of the problems that need to be addressed locally and in the elaboration of the solutions. Negotiations between knowledge produced in controlled conditions and the constraints imposed by local implementation conditions necessarily result into a form of program adaptation. Finally, a variety of social actors coming from a diversity of horizons, representing various interests, have to negotiate a common vision for the program as well as a course of action that takes into account the diversity of interests from relevant actors. All of this compose a process by which the different perspectives from the various actors are confronted in negotiations that redefine these perspectives and recompose existing networks. Public health and health promotion programs are not defined nor shaped solely by the logic models that translate expert knowledge into action but also through the actions of, and interactions between, the various actors located within the program's social space.

4.2. The Four Operations of Translation

Callon calls translation the ensemble of four operations that lead to the creation of new networks, or to the expansion of existing ones. This occurs through the integration of heterogeneous actors with different goals and interests, who are mobilized by common finalities and spokespersons with regards to a given situation (Callon, Lascoumes, & Barthe, 2001). These four operations that are called ·

---

[12] A case in point is the association between cigarette smoking and lung cancer. Nowadays, nobody would contest the scientific fact that cigarette smoking is a major cause of lung cancer. The heated controversy that involved leading statistician, epidemiologist and psychologist such as R. A. Fisher (1958a, 1958b), J. Berkson (1955) and H. J. Eysenck (Eysenck, Tarrant, & Woolf, 1960) in the 1950's concerning the association between cigarette smoking and lung cancer is almost forgotten now. See Vandenbroucke (1989), Stolley (1991) and the associated commentaries published in March 1st 1991 issue of the American Journal of Epidemiology for an interesting and informative debate about this controversy.

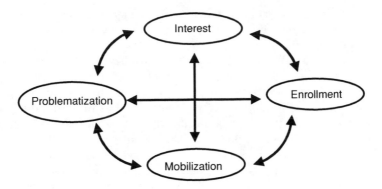

FIGURE 7.1. The four operations of translation.

problematization, interest, enrolment and mobilization[13], are iterative and do not necessarily follow a pre determined sequence as illustrated in Figure 7.1. The initiators of the translation process may vary. In most instances of public health programs, experts are leading the process, but documented cases exists where lay people have also initiated translation process by asking experts to help them find a solution to a situation they perceived as problematic and that required professional and scientific expertise. Finally, these operations do not presuppose a positive attitude of the initiator toward participatory approaches. These operations are merely milestones in a process.

The operation of problematization consists of identifying groups of relevant actors for a given issue, and in so doing, expanding the meaning of the issue. This operation is an acknowledgement that program initiators can only develop a limited understanding of the issue at hand and that they cannot control all aspects of the actions to be undertaken (Callon, Lascoume & Barthe, 2001). Groups of actors are deemed relevant, to the extent that they are perceived by the initiators as controlling resources or knowledge that are necessary for the full exploration of the question, or if they can give access to other relevant actors. To problematize a question is to demonstrate to the groups of relevant actors that the fulfilment of their own objectives and interests is linked to a given issue. Furthermore, the problematization operation is an essential step in mapping the social space of programs through establishing the social distances among the various relevant groups and between each of them and the issue of interest. In so doing it redefines various actors' beliefs about the question in an attempt to maximize the relevance of addressing this issue in the pursuit of their own objectives.

As an example of problematization, imagine that a group of local citizens (that we call initiators) conceive essentially as a moral issue attempts by municipal

---

[13] Callon's work is mainly published in French. The labels given of the four operations are those found in English translations of Callon's work. The original French labels are: problématisation, intéressement, enrôlement et déplacement.

authority to legalize street prostitution in their neighbourhood. If this is the case they are likely to initiate discussions with experts in ethics or with religious leaders and elaborate moral arguments in their confrontation with the proponents of this liberalisation. In an attempt to mobilize powerful allies they may revise this initial problematization so as to include the local public health authority as a significant actor. To do so, it is likely that they would have to alter the original meaning they ascribed to the legalization of prostitution and add a health dimension to it. This may lead them to hypothesize that there is an interest for public health authorities to preventing the possible dispersion of used condoms in parks and public spaces that may be associated with the legalization of prostitution[14]. The group of initiators could also formulate corresponding hypotheses regarding the local school authorities, adding to it an educational dimension and so on. In so doing however, they lose some of their own control over the definition of the problem and the actions to be undertaken regarding its solution. In reverse, failure to problematize relevant actors early in the action, may lead to the creation of a strong opposition that will elaborate its own problematization of the issue which may be conflicting. To problematize is to create associations between social actors and an issue of interest that is relevant in the pursuit of their own interests, elaborating a network among which some of the actors become essentials for the pursuit of the objectives and interests of other actors.

The operation of problematization can involve actors that are more or less active and more or less aware of their involvement in such a process[15]. Independently of their level of awareness, these groups of actors may behave according to the initiator's problematization explicitly or tacitly accepting the identity and role assigned to them or they may refuse this identity. The initiators need to engage in a negotiation with the groups of relevant actors in order to solidify the hypothetical relationships and identities hypothesised by the problematization. It is through the operation of interest that this negotiation develops.

Interest is the operation by which the initiators try to impose and to stabilize the other actors' role and identity in relation to the issue of interest through a series of mediated actions. The media is an apparatus the function of which is to allow the positioning of each group of actors in relationship with the question of interest (Akrich, Callon, & Latour, 1988a) To interest a group of actors is to establish with them a link, that may exclude other potential links. While problematization operations position the relevant actors with reference to a given social space,

---

[14] Note that the condom argument has acquired a strong health meaning mainly in association with the prevention of HIV-AIDS and Hepatitis C.

[15] In one of his early presentation of the theory of translation, Callon (1986) uses the example of a network composed of seashells, fishermen and scientists, in which each group needed the others in order for the particular seashell colony to continue to exist, for the fishermen to continue to earn their living by fishing from that colony, and the scientists to develop knowledge on that specific seashell specie. In this particular example, the scientists were the sole translators whereas the roles of the fishermen and of the seashells although as important, were more reactive than proactive.

interest sets up the content of their interaction with each other and more specifically with the issue of interest. Interest is based upon interpretations about what the other actors to be enrolled are and want. The interest apparatus is there to fix the identity of the actors in the network while interrupting competing relations, leading to the emergence of new social structures (Callon, 1986).

In the previous example, interest of the public health authority by the group of concerned citizens could develop through various apparatus and strategies. Citizens could alert the local newspapers and tell stories about children finding condoms in parks. They could invite physicians as speakers in citizens' assemblies. The reactions of the public health authorities to these various actions would in turn define the negotiation that would take place with the citizens. The public health authority could for example refuse to adopt the identity of a public regulatory authority embarking on a crusade against prostitution and adopt that of experts showing interest in structuring the experience of legalizing prostitution, and studying its consequence. The negotiation process that takes place with the interest operation may or may not transform the initial problematization.

The negotiations that take place during interest operation and that materialize the definitions and distributions of the various actors' roles are not always successful. Some actors may not behave as planned by the initiators, refusing their hypothetical identity. This identity can also be altered through the enrolment operation (Callon & Law, 1982). The operation of enrolment is the successful completion of an interest operation. " It designated the mechanism by which a role is defined and assigned to an actor who accepts it, thus integrating the network" (Callon, 1986). Enrolment strategies are numerous and various; they may follow a diversity of modalities and may occur simultaneously with a variety of actors. Once enrolled and their role redefined and accepted, groups of actors are part of a new network, their roles are coordinated in the pursuit of a common objective. As the system of action develops and new actors are identified as relevant, these roles are re-examined and redefined through iterative problematization and interest operations.

In our example, in their negotiation with the public health authorities, the group of citizens may have to accept that in order to count on this powerful ally, they would need to accept a modified version of the proposed legislation. For example, one in which the legalization is experimented in a well structured manner, which may suit better the long term objectives and mandate of a public health agency. This redefinition however implies also the redefinition of new roles for the sex workers and their relationships with the citizens, leading to a new problematization of the question in which new sex workers' identity would have to be entertained. The approval of these workers to enrol in such experimentation can only be obtained through another operation of interest, potentially led by the concerned citizens together with the public health authority.

The fourth operation is that of the mobilization of the actors. In all the operations of translation, the entirety of the individuals composing a group may not be involved throughout the translation process. In fact, most of the negotiations take place with mouthpieces whose legitimacy is denoted by their capacity to mobilize the group they represent. This mobilization of a group's interest by mouthpieces goes on until a limited number of actors can represent the whole network. The operation of mobilization is that by which selected actors identified as mouthpieces for the system or parts of it are entitled to, and do effectively, displace other actors enrolled. The capacity to mobilize a variety of actors in a network is thus the ultimate test of the legitimacy of a system's mouthpieces. The more heterogeneous and the less stable a network, the more intense the negotiation between the groups of actors to establish the legitimacy of the mouthpieces and the more likely it is that more than one mouthpiece will be necessary, or that the network will not survive the rise of a controversy. Of course, in highly hierarchical organisations, the legitimacy is often associated with the position in the hierarchy; however, in emerging networks where controversies are frequent, legitimacy is gained through a negotiation process. The legitimacy of the mouthpieces for those they represent can also be appraised though the various procedures that is required for the former to mobilize the latter. In our previous example because of the hierarchical and program structure of public health organisations, the professional responsible for AIDS prevention might be a representative spokesperson for this group of actors, and she will mobilize resources in her organisation by using the power associated with her role in this organisation, whereas for the group of sex workers, spokespersons may have to be designated through a consultative process. Even so, these spokespersons may have to have frequent meetings and discussions with the group they represent.

A translation process develops whenever social actors attempt to elaborate a novel network of relationships between various groups of actors who do not share *a priori* the same perspective and interests on an issue. Translation is the process by which these groups are strategically displaced in relation to each other and to an issue of interest. Translation is also the process by which a limited number of mouthpieces can express, in a common language, the will and discourse of the groups of actors involved in the network. A network of relationships between social actors is not static. New events, new actors or new relationships can contradict or shed doubts on the legitimacy of the mouthpieces or of their representation of the network, triggering controversies. The notion of dissidence describes the process of contesting the legitimacy of the mouthpieces by refusing the displacement and mobilization they call for. Callon calls "controversies" all those signs that show that mouthpieces legitimacy and capacity to mobilize the network is contested.

The translation process, as described by Callon, involves the constant adjustment of a plurality of actors in a social space through the operations of problematization, interest, enrolment, and mobilization of relevant actors (see Figure 7.1). As a social process, however, translation does not require that all actors from all groups act as translators of other groups of actors. Translators are those actors who initiate the translation process by: 1) problematizing a situation in terms of the roles and identities of relevant actors; 2) developing the media and apparatus to interest relevant actors; 3) enrolling other actors in their problematization and 4) mobilizing them into actions.

Translators can also act as network's mouthpieces and their legitimacy as mouthpieces is constructed throughout the translation process itself. Mouthpieces are successful translators of a given network, who can mobilize the network as well as represent it to outsiders.

4.3. Participation as a Multidirectional Translation Process

Translation, as described by Callon, is a series of operations in which each actor's level of activity and power is variable. As mentioned earlier, in his 1986 paper Callon uses as a case example a research program that involves three researchers, a fishermen union and a local seashell population. In this example, the researchers act as the sole translators and spokespersons for the whole network. Neither the seashells nor the fishermen took an active role in any of the translation operations; they reacted to the problematization, interest, enrolment and mobilization operated by researchers. These reactions with regards to the specific roles and identities assigned to them by the researchers' problematization often triggered negotiations and changes in the problematization, but neither the seashells nor the fisherman attempted to translate the other groups of actors in the pursuit of their interest. In addition, the specific seashells and fishermen enrolled in the process could be conceptualised as mouthpieces for their own groups. Not being actively involved in the translation however, neither the seashells nor the fishermen could or would constitute legitimate mouthpieces for the new network of relationships that was created by the translation process. One proposition is that although "translation" provides a valid and useful explanation of the social processes occurring in the social space of programs, translation is not equivalent to participation. In Callon's example, the researchers' control over the whole process was rarely challenged, and more importantly, these researchers were never translated by the other groups of actors. Neither seashells nor fishermen actively problematized the situation from their own perspective. As a result, translation as described in most of Callon's work is unidirectional. From the perspective of the translator the range of actions of the other actors is limited by the problematization operated by this unique translator. The main proposition of this chapter is that participation in health promotion programs occurs when at least two actors from different groups representing different initial interests are actively involved as translators of the other groups and as mouthpieces for the entire network. Participation is thus a multidirectional translation process.

Callon mostly reported on translation processes initiated, operated, and controlled by a single group of actors. Mostly concerned with knowledge production and socio-technical innovation, his work rarely addresses situations where scientists could not legitimately act as the sole translators for a given socio-technical network. I propose that participation is what happens when several groups among those involved in a social space develop their own problematization and initiate actions in order to translate other relevant groups. These multiple translation processes involve heterogeneous mouthpieces, each representing the problematization and interests of a relevant group of actors. Each translator is thus involved in two articulated translation processes. In one process, as spokespersons of a specific group of actors, they participate in the group's translation that they, as mouthpieces, can legitimately mobilize. In another process, in promoting the problematization and interests of their own group, they engage in active translations of other groups. Within this context, participation is the confrontation of various groups' problematization of a situation, where none of the groups can, or is willing to impose its own translation to the other groups.

These multiple translations need to be somewhat limited in number to occur in a specific space, otherwise the situation could be chaotic and the network may not mobilise a coherent set of actions. I thus propose that participation is characterised by a governing structure in which spokespersons from the various groups initiate translation operations and react to one another's translations in such a way that they can mobilize their own group when required and in a direction compatible with their network's interests and objectives. So, the multidirectional translation required in a participatory process entails a doubly articulated translation.

As illustrated in Figure 7.2, in the first level, a limited number of actors, who are mouthpieces for other actors, have to initiate a translation process among them. For that first-level translation to occur, the actors involved have to be engaged in a negotiation process in order to articulate the operations of the second-level translation in which their governance structure is engaged. This first level translation occurs within the governing structure and the second occurs between the governing structure and the other actors. The other level translation is occurring within and between each group's spokesperson and the groups they represent. They may or

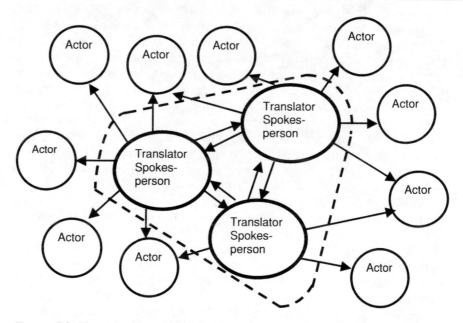

FIGURE 7.2. Network with multidirectional translations*.

* The single pointed arrows of this figure represent translators' capacity to mobilize other actors in the network.

may not be translators in their own group, but they need to be able to mobilise their groups in actions called for by the whole network's interests.

In such a doubly articulated network the mouthpieces assembled in the governing structure form a microcosm of the whole network whose capacity to create effective program space depends upon its capacity to anticipate the second level translation process as well as to imagine solutions to the problems that will be raised through iterative negotiations. Due to this, there is a constant reshaping of the program space to adapt to the ever changing results of the various negotiations is another characteristic of participatory programs. It is through this negotiation that participants to the governing structure map out a common problematization of all relevant groups of actors, including those that they are representing in the governing structure. One consequence of this process is the development of equivalences between their respective discourses and representations of the whole system. Each of the translator/spokesperson involved in the governing structure has the potential to become a legitimate spokesperson for the entire network while maintaining an obligation to remain a legitimate spokesperson of his or her own group of actors. The example presented in the Box below shows some of the explanatory power of framing participation in health promotion program as multidirectional translation.[16]

Many interesting features of the Kahnawake Schools Diabetes Prevention Project (KSDPP) acquire meaning when analysed through this multiple translation framework (see Macaulay et al., 1997; Potvin et al., 2003 for a detailed description of the project). This project identifies itself as a participatory project, founded upon the functional equal partnership between a group of academic researchers, a group of community researchers/professionals, and the community through the KSDPP Community Advisory Board (CAB), (Macaulay et al., 1998). An apparent paradox of this project is that despite the fact that most of the project's interventions are targeted at young people, the latter are not specifically mentioned in the "Code of Research Ethics" that form that partnership agreement, neither are they part of the governing structures of the project. The multidirectional articulation model of participation resolves this paradox. In their problematization of the situation of diabetes in their community, the group of elders and community leaders identified children and young people as a key group in the pursuit of their vision of a community free of diabetes. Community leaders could not however interest and enrol children with regards to diabetes prevention without the expert knowledge of community researchers and professionals. In addition, to have access to some of the required funds and

---

[16] In agreement with the Code of Research Ethics developed for this project (KSDPP, 2004), the chapter and the content of this box were discussed in a seminar with community researchers and representatives of the Community Advisory Board. The author of this chapter had been involved in this project as academic researcher for more than 10 years. Even if the information founding this example is all in the public domain, it was felt that such discussion was important to keep transparent all translation processes and all instances in which a program actor may be perceived as a potential spokesperson for the entire program.

resources, community leaders together with community researchers had to develop a research component; this was a necessary apparatus to interest funding agencies and mobilise their resources. This is why academic researchers were problematized, interested, and enrolled in the project. The community, through CAB as spokespersons, the community researchers/professionals and the academic researchers form the governing structure of translators for which the first level translation described earlier applies. Together, and in a concerted manner, they problematize, interest, enrol, and mobilize various other groups of actors, inside and outside of the community. The young people in the community form one such a group. They are mobilized through program activities and to the extent that CAB representatives and community staff in the governing structure are perceived as legitimate spokespersons of community young people's interest, there is no controversy and the governing structure can continue its work. Obviously, one could question whether program staff and community representatives are adequate spokespersons for community young people. The answer to that from a translation perspective is that a controversy will emerge when spokespersons will loose their legitimacy, signalling to the governing structure that the current problematization is not satisfactory for all actors involved and should be revised.

The double articulation that accompanies a multidirectional translation process also helps explain why some groups in the community may sense that their level of ownership over the project is low, despite its participatory nature (Cargo et al., 2003). Indeed, a longitudinal analysis of the sense of ownership over the project expressed by various groups in the community indicates that people in the Community Advisory Board together with the project staff, composed of community people, are the two groups with the greatest sense of ownership over all aspects of the project. Interestingly, the group of researchers from outside of the community express very little ownership about the intervention part of the project and a high satisfaction with that situation. In counterpart, some other community organisation members (referred to as community affiliates in Cargo et al. (2003)), who are associated with the development and implementation of some of the project's activities expressed low satisfaction with their actual level of control over the project. In terms of the two translation processes involved in this participatory program, these results indicate that the CAB members together with the program staff constitute the main actors in the translation process that occurs between the governing structure and community groups. The other community organisations that are translated by this governing structure have less control over the project. As for the academic researchers, their low level of perceived ownership over the project is an indication that the KSDPP has never been conceived as a hypothesis testing experiment and that they accept to be translated in the pursuit of community objectives. Their high level of satisfaction is a sign that through the project they can actively pursue academic objectives of conducting research, producing knowledge, and training graduate students (Potvin et al., 2003).

Finally, the doubly articulated translation creates a very dynamic space not only because each new compromise that results from the negotiation within the governing structure builds upon all previous negotiations, but also because these various iterations of the process transform the identity of all actors and therefore potentially affects the representativeness of the mouthpieces within the governing structure. This makes the whole situation much more complex and, more importantly, much more unstable than one characterized by a unique translator.

5. Health Promotion Programs, Uncertainty, and Participation

The complexity and dynamism resulting from participation in health promotion programs, conceived and experienced as a multidirectional translation process in a socio-technical network are key for the relevance of health promotion programs in reflexive modernity. Going back to uncertainty and individualization as two characteristics of reflexive modernity the remainder of this chapter will explore how participation allows health promotion programs to better cope with these features of our society.

Understanding health promotion programs as translation processes and participatory health promotion programs as multidirectional translation highlights two important features of participatory programs. The first is that programs are composed of social actors whose relationships are constantly negotiated within a dynamic problematization of the situation of interest. The second is that participation is a deliberate attempt to make problematization inclusive and relevant for a variety of groups of actors in the pursuit of their own objectives. These ideas are central to understanding how health promotion programs can orient social change in reflexive modernity.

A conception of health promotion programs that addresses the challenges of reflexive modernity should rest on the idea that in a reflexive world, a predictable chain of events leading to local transformations cannot be reliably triggered by implementing a program based upon universal knowledge. Meaning, programs cannot be reduced to technical solutions that can be imported in local contexts once they have proved effective. The working hypothesis that such a program could provide a valid answer to a local challenge needs to be problematized within an existing network of local actors. Such problematization, in turns, induces a translation process through which the meaning of the situation and the role of the various actors, including that of the program itself will be renegotiated. Adaptations to local contexts and realignments of the planned actions have to be negotiated continuously because any program aims at a moving target, and the target is moving precisely as a result of the events associated with the program. By proposing a novel problematization of a given situation, health promotion programs introduce new meanings and roles, the effect of which is to induce a new dynamism in the situation of interest. Independently of the carefulness of the planning process, health promotion programs not only are operating in uncertainty but they are themselves sources of uncertainty.

There are three possible reactions to this state of affair. The optimist modernist reaction is to deny that programs contribute in creating a more complex reality and that when appropriately manipulated, technical solutions derived from objective science leads to predictable outcomes. The pessimist modernist reaction is mainly associated with post modernism; and rests upon the thought that scientific knowledge cannot be translated into technical innovations with predictable effects; there is no possibility to deliberately orient social change in the pursuit of specific objectives. A third posture is to attempt to manage this uncertainty associated with the implementation of health promotion programs. One way of doing so is to foster participation by inviting a variety of groups of relevant actors to actively engage in their own problematization of the situation and to render the multidirectional translation that characterize the process as transparent as possible through a governance structure made of spokespersons of the various groups actively involved as translators.

Uncertainty does not mean that the future is opaque and that anything could happen. Quite on the contrary, it refers to situations in which the range of plausible future developments is identifiable but where each of these possible futures cannot be assigned an exact probability of occurrence. I contend that participation helps manage this uncertainty and this in two ways. Firstly, the exploration of a wider range of possible futures through the negotiation and confrontation of the problematization that various groups of actors entertain about the situation provides a richer and more comprehensive assessment of the mechanism that produced any given situation, therefore resulting in a better informed action. Secondly, because the simultaneous occurrence of those multiple problematizations necessitates the constitution of functioning governance structures that rest on the involvement of spokespersons, a greater variety of groups of relevant actors can be mobilized through the program, thus resulting in a greater capacity to make things happen.

6. Conclusion

This chapter used Callon's sociology of translation to theorize public participation in health promotion and public health programs. In so doing, it illustrated how social theory may be put at work to better understand a key health promotion practice. More than that, by linking a macro social theory such as that of reflexive modernity to a micro social theory of action like the sociology of translation it is expected that such a theoretical exercise would lead to a critical appraisal of public participation as a practice, justifying its promotion in specific situations and providing health promotion practitioners with practical ideas on how to facilitate participation.

The problem, this chapter argues in line with Giddens' conception of modernity, is that the increasingly reflexive nature of our world renders the applications in local context of solutions derived from universal knowledge more and more problematic. This is even more so when social processes are involved because this is where reflexivity is primarily at play, and as such, probably the reason why the need to advance public participation was more acute in health promotion than in health care for example, because the health promotion clearly positions health in the social domain. In addition, dealing with local social contexts for program implementation necessarily entails some degree of uncertainty, even for programs that are widely recognized as effective. Nonetheless, one should never consider public participation lightly and simply. The uncritical definition of public participation as the involvement of all concerned actors in all aspects of the program is plainly untenable and leads potentially to complete chaos.

Understanding public participation as a multidirectional translation process puts the emphasis on the negotiation process that needs to take place between representative and legitimate spokespersons of the various groups of actors. While these actors may problematize the situation differently, their mobilization is crucial for exploring and pursuing the actualisation of locally relevant scenarios. So, there are various degrees of public participation both in terms in the variety and heterogeneity of groups of actors actively involved as translators. In addition, there are varying degrees in terms of the power and legitimacy of the groups' spokespersons in the program's governance structure.

In closing, health promotion must be conceived, at least in part, as a practice that advances public health's capacity to fulfil its public responsibility. Its ability to do so, however, is not linked to the power of its ideology but to its profound and critical understanding of how those practices that are its trademark, such as participation, operate and contribute to improving the public's health in our contemporary society.

References

Akrich, M., Callon, M., & Latour, B. (1988a, Juin). A quoi tient le succès des innovations. .Premier épisode: l'art de l'intéressement. *Annales des mines. Gérer et comprendre, 12,* 4–17.

Akrich, M., Callon, M., & Latour, B. (1988b, Septembre). A quoi tient le succès des innovations. Deuxième épisode: l'art de choisir les bons porte-parlole. *Annales des mines. Gérer et comprendre, 12,* 18–29.

Arnstein, S. R. (1969). A ladder of citizen participation. *Journal of the American Institute of Planners, 35*(4), 216–224.

Beck, U. (1992). *Risk society: Towards a new modernity.* London: Sage.

Beck, U. (1994). The reinvention of politics: Toward a theory of reflexive modernization. In U. Beck, A. Giddens, & S. Lash (Eds.), *Reflexive modernization. Politics, traditions and aesthetics in the modern social order* (pp. 1–55). Stanford, CA: Stanford University Press.

Beck, U. (2000). Risk society revisited. In B. Adam, U. Beck, & J. Van Loon (Eds.), *The risk society and beyond. Critical issues for social theory* (pp. 221–229). London: Sage.

Beck, U., Giddens, A., & Lash, S. (Eds.). (1994). *Reflexive modernization. Politics, traditions and aesthetics in the modern social order.* Stanford, CA: Stanford University Press.

Berkson, J. (1955). The statistical study of association between smoking and lung cancer. *Mayo Clinic Proceedings, 30,* 319–347.

Bisset, S. L., Cargo, M., Delormier, et al. (2004). Legitimising diabetes as a community health issue: A care analysis of the Kahnawake Schools Diabetes Prevention project. *Health Promotion International, 19,* 317–326.

Callon, M. (1986). Elements pour une sociologie de la traduction. La domestication des coquilles Saint-Jacques et des marins-pêcheurs dans la baie de Saint-Brieuc. *L'année sociologique, 36*, 169–208.

Callon, M. (1989a). Introduction. In M. Callon (Ed.), *La science et ses réseaux. Genèse et circulation des faits scientifiques* (pp. 7–33). Paris: La découverte.

Callon, M. (1989b). L'agonie d'un laboratoire. In M. Callon (Ed.), *La science et ses réseaux. Genèse et circulation des faits scientifiques* (pp. 173–214). Paris: La découverte.

Callon, M. (1999). Le réseau comme forme émergente et comme modalité de coordination: le cas des interactions stratégiques entre firmes industrielles et laboratoires académiques. In M. Callon, P. Cohendet, N. Curien, J.-M. Dalle, F. Eymard-Duvernay, D. Foray, & E. Schenk (Eds.), *Réseau et coordination* (pp. 13–64). Paris: Economica.

Callon, M. (2001). Actor network theory. In N. Smelster & P. Balste (Eds.), *International encyclopedia of the social and behavioral sciences* (pp. 62–66). Oxford, UK: Pergamon.

Callon, M., Lascoumes, P., & Barthe, Y. (2001). *Agir dans un monde incertain. Essaie sur la démocratie technique.* Paris: Seuil.

Callon, M., & Latour, B. (1991). Introduction. In M. Callon, & B. Latour (Eds.), *La science telle qu'elle se fait* (pp. 7–36). Paris: La découverte.

Cargo, M., Levesque, L., Macaulay, A. C., et al., with the KSDPP Comunity Advisory Board. (2003). Community governance of the Kahnawake Schools Diabetes Prevention Project, Kahnawake Territory, Mohawk Nation, Canada. *Health Promotion International, 18*, 177–187.

COMMIT Research Group. (1991). Community Intervention Trial for Smoking Cessation (COMMIT): Summary of design and intervention. *Journal of the National Cancer Institute, 83*, 1620–1628.

Contandripoulos, D. (2004). A sociological perspective on public participation in health care. *Social Science & Medicine, 58*, 321–330.

Eysenk, H. J., Tarrant, M., & Woolf, M. (1960). Smoking and personality. *British Medical Journal, 1*, 1456–1460.

Fassin, D. (1996). *L'espace politique de la santé.* Paris: Presses universitaires de France.

Fisher, R. A. (1958a). Lung cancer and cigarettes? (Letter). *Nature, 182*, 108.

Fisher, R. A. (1958b). Cancer and smoking (Letter). *Nature, 182*, 596.

Fournier, P., & Potvin, L. (1995). Participation communautaire et programmes de santé: les fondements du dogme. *Sciences sociales et santé, 13*, 39–59.

Frenk, J., Bobadilla, J.-L., Stern, C., et al. (1994). Elements of a theory of health transition. In L. C. Chen, A. Kleinman, & N. C. Ware (Eds.), *Health and social change in international perspective* (pp. 25–49). Boston: Harvard University Press.

Giddens, A. (1990). *The consequences of modernity.* Stanford, CA: Stanford University Press.

Giddens, A. (1994). Living in a post-traditional society. In U. Beck, A. Giddens, & S. Lash (Eds.), *Reflexive modernization. Politics, traditions and aesthetics in the modern social order* (pp. 56–109). Stanford, CA: Stanford University Press.

Green, L. W., George, M. A., Daniel, M., et al. (1995). *Study of participatory research in health promotion: Review and recommendations for the development of participatory research in health promotion in Canada.* Ottawa: The Royal Society of Canada.

Green, L. W., & Kreuter, M. (1999). *Health promotion planning: An educational and ecological approach.* Mountain View, CA: Mayfield.

Green, L. W., & Mercer, S. (2001). Can public health researchers and agencies reconcile the push from funding bodies and pull from communities. *American Journal of Public Health, 91*, 1926–1929.

Illich, I. (1975). *Limits to medicine. Medical nemesis: The expropriation of health*. London, UK: McClelland & Stewart.

Lash, S. (1999). *Another modernity a different rationality*. Oxford: Blackwell.

Latour, B. (1989). *La science en action*. Paris: La découverte.

Latour, B. (1991). *Nous n'avons jamais été modernes: essai d'anthropologie symétrique*. Paris: La découverte.

Latour, B. (1999). *Politiques de la nature. Comment faire entrer les sciences dans la démocratie*. Paris: La découverte.

Lefebvre, R. C., Lasater, T. M., Carleton, R. A., et al. (1987). Theory and delivery of health programming in the community: The Pawtucket Heart Health Program. *Preventive Medicine, 16*, 80–95.

Macaulay, A. C., Delormier, T., McComber, A. M., et al. (1998). Participatory research with Native community of Kahnawake creates innovative Code of Research Ethics. *Canadian Journal of Public Health, 89*, 105–108.

Macaulay, A.C., Paradis, G., Potvin, L., et al. (1997). The Kahnawake Schools Diabetes Prevention Project: A diabetes primary prevention program in a native community in Canada. Intervention and baseline results. *Preventive Medicine, 26*, 779–790.

MacKian, S., Elliott, H., Busby, H., et al. (2003). "Everywhere and nowhere": Locating and understanding the "new" public health. *Health & Place, 9*, 219–229.

Nutbeam, D., Smith, C., & Catford, J. (1990). Evaluation in health education: A review of progress, possibilities and problems. *Journal of Epidemiology and Community Health, 44*, 83–89.

Potvin, L. (2004). On the nature of programs: Health promotion programmes as action. *Cienca, & Saude Coletiva, 9*, 731–738.

Potvin, L., Cargo, M., McComber, et al. (2003). Implementing participatory intervention and research in communities: Lessons from the Kahnawake Schools Diabetes Prevention Project. *Social Science & Medicine, 56*, 1295–1305.

Potvin, L., & Chabot, P. (2002). Splendour and misery of epidemiology for evaluation of health promotion. *Revista Brasileira de Epidemiologia, 5*(suppl. 1), 91–103.

Potvin, L., Gendron, S., Bilodeau, A., & Chabot, P. (2005). Integrating social science theory into public health practice. *American Journal of Public Health, 95*, 591–595.

Potvin, L., Haddad, S., & Frohlich, K. L. (2001). *Beyond process and outcome evaluation: A comprehensive approach for evaluating health promotion programmes*. In I. Rootman, M. Goodstadt, B. Hyndman, D.V. McQueen, L. Potvin, J. Springett, & E. Ziglio (Eds.), *Evaluation in health promotion. Principles and perspectives* (pp. 45–62). Copenhague: WHO Regional Publications. European series No. 92.

Rifkin, S. B., Muller, F., & Bichmann, W. (1988). Primary health care: On measuring participation. *Social Science & Medicine, 26*, 931–940.

Robertson, A., & Minkler, M. (1994). New health promotion movement: A critical examination. *Health Education Quarterly, 21*, 295–312.

Rootman, I., Goodstadt, M., Potvin, L., & Springett, J. (2001). A framework for health promotion evaluation. In I. Rootman, M. Goodstadt, B. Hyndman, D. V. McQueen, L. Potvin, J. Springett, & E. Ziglio (Eds.), *Evaluation in health promotion: Principles and perspectives* (pp. 7–38). Copenhague: WHO Regional Publications. European series No. 92.

Salonen, J. T., Kottke, T. E., Jacobs, D. R., & Hannan, P. J. (1986). Analysis of community-based cardiovascular disease prevention studies—evaluation issues in the North Karelia Project and the Minnesota Heart Health Program. *International Journal of Epidemiology, 15*, 176–182.

Scheirer, M. A. (1994). Designing and using process evaluation. In J. S. Wholey, H. P. Hatry, & K. E. Newcomer (Eds.), *Handbook of practical program evaluation* (pp. 40–68). San Francisco: Jossey-Bass.

Stolley, P. D. (1991). When genius errs: R. A. Fisher and the lung cancer controversy. *American Journal of Epidemiology, 133*, 416–425.

Vandenbroucke, J. P. (1989). Those who were wrong. *American Journal of Epidemiology, 130*, 3–5.

White, D. (2000). Consumer and community participation: A reassessment of process, impact, and value. In G. L. Albrecht, R. Fitzpatrick, & S. C. Scrimshaw (Eds.), *The handbook of social studies in health & medicine* (pp. 465–480). Thousand Oaks, CA: Sage.

Zakus, J. D. L., & Lysack, C. L. (1998). Revisiting community participation. *Health Policy and Planning, 13*, 1–12.

8
Thinking Health Promotion Sociologically

LAURA BALBO

1. Introduction

Processes of social change in both the scientific domain and in society -hence, also in people's everyday practices—are in many ways interrelated.

Referring to the "third public health revolution"[1] Kickbusch argues that its "timing ... is not incidental and linked purely to scientific progress but ... it coincides with a revolution in the overall organization of our societies". She further explains that "the major restructuring of late modern societies" and the development of sociological theories which focus upon circumstances, processes and transformations can be seen as *consequences of modernity.* (Giddens, 1990)

Another approach to understanding how recent developments in both the social and health sciences are linked may also be addressed from the perspective of *"thinking scientific practices and theories sociologically"*, as suggested by Pierre Bourdieu[2]. I would argue that it appears of great interest to analyze the point in time when theories of "modernity" and the "third public health revolution" converge. It is this chapter's intent to describe modernity and its consequences as an overall scenario, or "frame"[3], and suggest that a number of such consequences are crucial for the legitimization and development of health promotion as a paradigm, a shared culture in contemporary society, a set of practices in everyday life.

My main point is that health promotion is made possible, and in fact supported by the social circumstances of modernity. It is with this focus that I see the following discussion as an exercise in "thinking health promotion sociologically".

Anthony Giddens has described the process of change using the terms *detraditionalization* and *reflexive modernization:* both the concept and the experience

---

[1] This definition was first put forward by Lester Breslow (1999). In her chapter Ilona Kickbusch analyzes how this concept has been developed in subsequent contributions.
[2] *Penser sociologiquement*, as Bourdieu suggests, means "permettre à ceux qui font la science de mieux comprendre les méchanisms sociaux qui orientent la pratique scientifique ... soumettre la science à une analyse historique et sociologique ... " (Bourdieu, 2001, p. 8). Also Bourdieu, 1997.
[3] The use of the term "frame" as suggested by Lakoff (2004) is of great pertinence here.

of health have been deeply transformed. There has been a shift from fighting illness to promoting practices which prevent or delay illness; from highly specific measures of diagnosis and therapy to general issues concerning the environment, the economy, urban living, organizational practices, and education, which in turn affects the health and quality of life for all. While these are typical areas of policy-making and political governance, they also translate into personal, political and social decisions of everyday life. In fact in modernity positive health and well-being are basic aims (and responsibilities) of individual, familial, and community practices.

Keeping healthy is no longer considered to belong only in the realm of the "sacred", as it was the case in the past, totally under control of supernatural agents. Circumstances of life and death, issues of basic rights, the culture of society as a whole are involved. Not only strategic behavior and rationality, deep-seated emotions and feelings have come to be considered.

While it is clearly not the aim of the present discussion to address all aspects of the social change theories which deal with modernity[4]. I believe it is important to discuss the complexity of the health discourse of the present situation, properly analyzing all of its components. Health as "a resource for living" as Lester Breslow (Breslow, 1999) put it or as I would like to argue, health practices as they are addressed in the health promotion platform are defined not as individual lifestyles and personal strategies, but as a culture of shared values of healthy living and well-being; practices which comprise an integral part of our daily life experience in modernity.

Starting with Giddens' theoretical discussion of *reflexivity* and *agency* in modernity or in other words traits of competence, skills, and learning which characterize modern society (Giddens1990, 1991), I shall insist on two further developments. First, to introduce elements of uncertainty, risk, and insecurity as crucial issues in the debate about globalization (Anthony Giddens himself, Zygmut Bauman, Ulrich Beck, Robert Castel, Robert Lash, Alberto Melucci). The second is the *gender perspective*, as it has been increasingly legitimized in recent years in a most valuable literature. I argue that women's (or as I rather prefer to say, adult women's) roles and responsibilities in day-by-day arrangements require agency, reflexivity and lifelong learning: such traits are of crucial relevance for the social functioning of modernity (M.C. Bateson, 1995; L. Balbo, 2004).

The processes I have mentioned—which characterize all aspects of contemporary life—are no doubt particularly visible in the health discourse. No longer patients, rather social actors, or citizens in general, relevant in the health field. Practices defined as *health literacy* and *health competence*, investing in health, as well as a variety of health-producing experiences, participation in health-promoting

---

[4] For a comprehensive discussion of the "sociologies of modernity" see Martuccelli, 1999. "Late modernity" (Giddens); "second-modernity" and "new modernity" (Beck); "*surmodernité* " (Balandier, Augé), *pleine modernité* (Touraine) are other well-established definitions.

projects or forums, will be addressed. Lay knowledge and lay participation as such are in fact "consequences of modernity".

In order to connect the theoretical analysis of modernity with the aims of understanding ongoing societal processes, many unresolved questions concerning concrete life conditions need to be discussed. A few of the many relevant issues will accordingly be introduced, the following three in particular.

First, the divide in contemporary society between those who are secure or well-off and those who are "excluded" because of persisting, actually increasing, inequities in access to material resources, public services and information is obviously crucial to the analysis presented here; this includes social class, gender, race and ethnicity. Secondly, in emphasizing traits of "self-reflexivity" and "lifelong-learning" in people's daily living and what I shall refer to as "critical learning", the role of the media and the enormous power of systems of communication must be considered.

Finally I will address economic interests and profit mechanisms as related to the field of health. Health promotion is located within this context. The dimensions of inequality and complexity become central to our discussion.

2. Redefining Modernity

I see the shift to a "post—traditional order" or a "de-traditionalized society" as an appropriate background to the present discussion (Giddens, 1991). In describing this shift Giddens argues that the "balance" between tradition and modernity—in what he defines as "reflexive modernization"—has been dramatically altered. He considers crucial the need for the social sciences today to "face a new agenda . . . the emergence of a post-traditional society" (Giddens, 1994).

A shift is to be noticed from concepts such as reflexivity, knowledge-accumulation, rationality, to the growing focus on (and concern with) ours as a "risk society" (Beck, 1993, 2002), a "society of uncertainty"[5] (Bauman, 1998). In the *risk society* one is faced with the unexpected and the non-rational (Hake, 1998; Morin, 2000; Dupont, 2003). Robert Castel (2003) points to two specific components in this process: on the one hand the increasing weakness of the previous system of social protection, hence, "la remontée de l'insecurité sociale"; on the other the emergence of risks that traditional institutional agencies are not prepared to deal with.

In fact "risk" in its many forms is to be taken as a permanent component in the development of the new global order (and in people's everyday life). What is argued is that a "new culture, a culture of uncertainty" and social and personal coping skills are needed, that may enable us to "deal with ambivalence" and to "govern risk". In the process there are however "winners and losers" (Giddens, 1990): in the face of growing complexity and unpredictability many just cannot cope with the highly

---

[5] "Insecurity" and hence "uncertainty", *Sichereit* and *Unsichereit,* are Bauman's terms.

demanding circumstances of such a system and the challenges they are expected to meet. Increasingly, attitudes of fundamentalism, pressing demands for simple answers emerge in all areas of society and spheres of human behavior.

The concept of "chaos" has also been introduced. What was until recently taken for granted (firmly established expectations and appropriate, reflexive strategies) makes little sense under newly emerging conditions. "Le reve de securité totale", our dream of leading our lives in totally secure circumstances—which emerged in western societies in previous decades—no longer holds (Castel, 2003).

In a similar vein Jane Jacobs (Jacobs, 2004, p.14) describes the collapse of "strong and successful cultures caused by assault from within". The world faces unpredictable effects related to environmental risks and trends in the global economy (transnational migrations, mass poverty), wars and terrorism. Technological innovation and developments in scientific research introduce previously unconceivable experiments related to human life, and death, and the choices which they imply; threatening diseases spread across nations (Barry, 2004).

3. The Learning Experience: Redefining Education and Learning

I want to once again stress how the elements described as self-reflexivity, access to information, competence building, and learning, are central to the present analysis. These are of such relevance to my argument that I hope it will be considered acceptable to dwell on a number of contributions in this area. These, I would argue, help to clarify how the focus which has been chosen in this chapter is appropriate in updating our discussion of health promotion.

Considering the learning dimension at all levels of the social system, including actors in everyday life, has been a major contribution in Giddens' definition of "reflexive modernization". One "can never be sure that any given element of ... knowledge will not be revised". (Giddens, 1990, pp. 38–39). Social practices, he argues, "are constantly examined and reformed in the light of incoming information about those very practices ... " Social actors[6] are described as competent, informed, and knowledgeable: in fact they constantly engage in building their social knowledge and putting it to use.

Reflexive social practices characterize society, human action, individuals as well as institutions and organizations. Actors at all levels are capable of, and required to, pursue such practices. The dimension of everyday life becomes central.

"We are all caught up ... in a grand experiment ... The global experiment of modernity intersects with, and influences as it is influenced by, the penetration of modern institutions

---

[6] "Social actors", as this concept is understood in this chapter, also refers to the *sociologie du Sujet,* a theoretical approach which has been central in Alain Touraine's thinking. See in particular, Touraine 1992; Touraine and Khosrokhavar, 2000. In my discussion however I do not use this concept with a "gender-blind" approach but I shall insist on the role of women in the functioning of everyday life and in health practices in particular.

into the tissue of day-by-day life ... Everyday experiments concern some very fundamental issue of self and identity, but they also involve a multiplicity of changes and adaptations in daily life." (Giddens, 1994, 59, 60)

Within this context, Giddens adds, "we have no choice but to choose how to live and how to act" and this points to elements of opportunity (in fact, of freedom) in modernity, as well as related responsibility.

I would like to stress how practices of "reflexive accumulation", or in slightly different words, "continuous learning", "lifelong learning" are required in, as well as made possible by, daily experiences. These aspects are central to my discussion of health and well being and I take them to be crucial components in what will be described as the scenario of a health culture.

The ongoing theoretical and political debate on contemporary society as a knowledge-based society or a learning-based society helps to set the background to what I emphasize and refer to developments both in the scholarly community and in public and policy discourse. In synthesizing a few of the many lines of reasoning that I take to be relevant the main shift in paradigm is from the concern with learning and education, as located in the early years of life and taking place in the context of specialized institutions, to continuous, lifelong learning. It is important to consider a variety of related contexts, working life being a primary setting, but not the only one, and a variety of practices ("learning by doing, using, and interacting" as Bengt-Abe Lundvall recently suggested (Lundvall, 2004). "Practical learning" is also a useful addition to how I would define *lifelong learning* in circumstances of modernity.

All components of the social system are involved: individuals in their daily lives, civil society in the widest sense, the institutional apparatus and a variety of organizations, the private as well as the public sector.

In the early sixties Jerome Bruner made the suggestion that there is "a modern mind" and introduced his redefinition of knowing and learning as "a multidimensional process". We hence came to consider the process of "learning to learn", and outstanding social scientists (Bateson, Gardner, Habermas, Luhmann, Morin) entered this theoretical debate from multiple perspectives. A most relevant contribution is the principle of learning "to un-learn", which is also included in what Giddens defines as "reflexive appropriation of knowledge": not a "zero-sum game" as Jerome Bruner remarks (Bruner, 1996).

I now briefly turn to a set of different contributions included at present in a variety of E.U. initiatives, which address processes in our "information society" or "société de la communication". The pressure of global competition and related issues of innovation and institution-building sets the background for a new agenda, projects and policies aimed at investing in learning as a pre-requisite for the "information and knowledge-based economy and society"[7].

---

[7] Jacques Delors' path-breaking policy commitment in 1993 is of course of primary importance. Reference ought also be made to the 1996 Green paper "Living and Working in the Information Society" and, following the Lisbon Treaty in 2000, to the term

The "White Paper on Teaching and Learning" issued in 1995 and several subsequent documents focus on adult, lifelong learning: hence on innovative practices of training and knowledge-formation, seen as necessary requirements in the perspective of a globally competitive workforce, but also as values of equity and democracy. What I wish to emphasize is the shift from the prevailing emphasis on making the economic system more adequate to challenges of international competition and innovation to considering the performance of a society as a whole. The issue now is how to take the learning dimension to all levels of the system. The systemic, dynamic elements have come to the fore. Learning is seen as "a public good" ("*bien public*": Gorz, 2003). Competence and learning in the health experience are obviously of crucial relevance. Empowering experiences also characterize our times: we need to be aware of the fact that in reflexive modernization "enabling conditions" and "elements of constraint" coexist (Giddens and Lash, 1997).

4. Adult Women and Lifelong Learning

I argue that introducing a gender perspective and more specifically focusing on adult women as social actors adds to the predominantly gender and generation-blind understanding of the concepts we have considered so far: de-traditionalization, reflexive modernization, the learning-based society. This in fact I see as a particularly appropriate element in our effort at thinking health and health promotion sociologically. I shall draw on Mary Catherine Bateson's description of women's life as "a work in progress", pointing to their "multiple beginnings" and "discontinuous lives", and to practices of "improvisation" (M.C. Bateson, 1990):

"Ongoing improvisations are required . . . and this is to be seen as an emergent pattern rather than as an aberration . . . composing a life is what we all, in the reality in which we live, are called upon to accomplish . . . "(pp. 232–233)

Precisely because of their living with multiple obligations, adult women are likely to develop a particularly favorable attitude to "improvising", as well as to "self-interpreting and self-monitoring" as Mary Catherine Bateson indicates. In my own research I have described the impact of conditions of modernity on adult women, pointing to their "quilt-making" practices in the organization of daily living and their need to develop skills of reflexivity and learning[8].

Being able to *adjust* to what is considered to be appropriate under changing conditions—and to *dis-adjust* as well—constantly re-assessing solutions and

---

"knowledge-society" which set this as a E.U. objective in research and policy initiatives. Yet another objective is a "Europe-wide learning society" (OECD 2000). *Lifelong learning* hints at the deep-reaching demographic transformations and changed life-course patterns as well as at more general social and cultural traits in "our modernity. A recent Report (*Adult Continuing Education,* CEDE, 2003) indicates that presently a higher number of adult persons than children and youngsters are involved in education and training activities.

[8] This I have argued on several occasions. See in particular Balbo 2004.

arrangements ("self-accounting" is Bruner's term): this is how learning in the context of modernity is to be described. It obviously concerns men as well as women and different generations in different ways.

In addressing issues of health and well-being it seems reasonable to focus on adult women: it is women who primarily are in charge. In fact they perform a great part of the required activities and do much of the necessary learning. Due to overall societal trends in recent decades and transformations in daily living, adult women have re-defined their roles and adjusted to expectations which are increasingly demanding in terms of time organization and skills (Lallement, 2003). This holds true for their professional activities of course, for their choices as clients of public services and as consumers, and in daily housekeeping tasks. Furthermore, far from being experiences of passive accumulation and of isolated, lonely, private efforts, these take place in a variety of "public" contexts: women do networking, they are the majority of those participating in social movements and grassroot activities, and with increasing visibility they play the role of spokespersons for advocacy initiatives. Considering practices of healthy living and wellness it is expected of women that they develop appropriate competences and acquire what is often highly specialized information. Responsibility for their own health as well as for the well-being and health of family members (child-rearing of course, and how to face the complex needs of those who are sick or aging) is a major component of women's social roles[9].

A crucial aspect is coping with often contradictory flows of information. One example in recent years is the controversial evidence on risks involved in the generalized use of hormone replacement therapies for symptoms of menopause: following the 2002 publication of the U.S. National Institute of Health Report "Women's Health Initiative" and a massive media campaign, a great many women decided to drop the therapy, the numbers going from 15 million down to 9 million users in one year in the United States only. Newly acquired scientific discoveries are communicated to the lay public at an increasingly rapid rhythm. Moreover, quality care and user-friendly health services, hopefully positive implications of technological and scientific innovations are sought. Continuous learning is required on such diverse aspects as eating habits and smoking, chronic illnesses and disabilities, rare diseases; depression and mental health.

5. Daily Practices, Health, and Wellness

One interesting aspect is the widespread interest in "non-conventional" medicine. In the context of what is now a global market and of global communication networks, an extraordinary variety of options are offered, ranging from homeopathy

---

[9] A Report from the European Foundation for the Improvement of Living and Working Conditions (2004, www.eurofound.eu.int/publications/EF03107.htm) covering twenty-eight European countries indicates that "on average, 25% of respondents ... provide continuous care to someone with a long-term illness or disability".

to acupuncture to herbs to what have come to be defined as mind-body techniques, all the way to hypnosis and meditation.

Recent figures indicate that persons living in western countries have greater than before access to a variety of choices in health care, and are turning to alternative or complementary remedies[10]. It is also a fact that transnational migrations and "diaspora communities", inasmuch as they make it possible for great numbers of persons in these communities to remain in touch with their cultures and practices, contribute to a less homogeneous and less west-centered scenario of therapies and remedies.

In this perspective the relevance of the process which has been defined the "feminization of migration" (Castles and Miller, 1998) also ought to be mentioned. It has been indicated that because of their family obligations, more than it is the case for men, adult women in migration establish relations with social services, schools, and health agencies in the countries of arrival. In their roles as "nannies and maids" (Ehrenreich and Russel Hochschild, 2003) they learn "western" wellness and health practices; while at the same time they introduce these back in their own countries ("traditional" health practices also are exported, put to test, re-defined). Issues of care and love, as Ehrenreich and Russel Hochschild argue, are "exported" transnationally. Health care styles and learning processes concerning health ought to be considered in the same perspective.

Concepts referring to previously unknown conditions help to clarify the point I am trying to make, such as *les patients auto-soignants* (Documentation Française, 1993); the "internet informed patient"; "e-health".

An enormously increased amount of information concerning research, therapies, and remedies is now made available through the internet. In fact, not information only, a growing number of medical products are available *on-line*, and web sites promoting and selling health products proliferate. Patients and caregivers, both professionals and non-professionals, in fact the great majority of people in their daily experience are, and need to be, informed, competent, active social actors. Continuously developing technologies make home-care and self-care possible. Hence, patients and their caregivers need to be knowledgeable about the diagnostic as well as the medical equipment which are currently used.

Something also needs to be said about practices of self-medication and of the enormous use, in the U.S. particularly, of "over the counter products"[11].

---

[10] It has been reported that nearly half of all adults in the United States go outside the health system for some of their care; in other words, they consider "integrative care" practices and "complementary therapies" as additional, or alternative remedies. The figure which has been given indicates some 600 million visits a year to non-conventional healers in the U.S.; in Europe, sales of homeopathic cures for last year are estimated to top 3 billion (*Newsweek*, December 2, 2002; WHO, 2002; Eisenberg & al., 1998). A WHO Report suggests that in France and Germany 75% of the population make use of "alternative" remedies or therapies (*Le Monde Diplomatique*, September 2001).

[11] "Be MedWise" is a campaign launched in 2002 by the National Council on Patient Information and Education, aiming at promoting responsible self- medication. Data (collected in 2001) on the level of patients' information have been published by the Consumer Healthcare

Psychotherapy and counseling, activities within voluntary associations and self-help groups are part of the picture. The fact that choices concerning sexual life and reproduction, death and dying, are no longer kept within the "private sphere" of people's lives is of extraordinary relevance. Again women in particular are expected to be producers and users of relevant knowledge and know-how. Choosing among an unprecedented number of alternative options, being properly advised about available solutions, making decisions as to coping strategies: these are major responsibilities in the organization of people's daily life. Constantly updating and evaluating one's knowledge and information in the health field is required.

Let me consider again a point which was made earlier to address the primary question of this discussion: in the process of modernization the concept as well as the experience of health has been transformed. How health in our overall culture (and in everyday practices as well) has come to be what it now is, is in fact a major component of the picture.

The crucial transformation is due to the fact that medical competence and knowledge no longer belong to a "world apart", a completely separate sphere of social organization and daily life.

As Giddens states,

"Our relationship to science and technology today is different from that characteristic of earlier times ... Lay people "took" opinions from the experts. The more science and technology intrude into our lives ... the less this perspective holds." (1994, p. 31)

It appears indeed that most people no longer are willing to accept rules that were until very recently taken for granted. Though it is true that the doctor/ patient relationship is still strongly asymmetrical (in certain circumstances at least) it is often the case that patients or clients, or those who are their caregivers, are well-informed: hence they are in a position to negotiate or choose with regard to treatments and therapies. The fact that the medical profession is at risk of, and in fact, well-insured against, possible claims on the part of those attended to, confirms the shifts in trust and power. In the health field in fact there has been a dramatic shift affecting relations of authority, trust and legitimization between doctors and their patients as well as the official health system and everyday health practices, "self-reliance" being one way to define this trend. In short: the distinction between producers and users of health has become blurred.

The expression *health promotion* itself is grounded on people's daily practices (Kickbush, 2003). *Learning*, updating information and constantly re-assessing everyday life choices and arrangements, is obviously part of this process.

The "consequences of modernity" and open issues: communication, complexity, inequality, learning, information, competence are abstract terms unless we take into account how these relate to other components of the everyday living experience.

Products Association: 79% of the medical personnel interviewed consider consumers to be inadequately informed about the products they use.

Communication and information processes in the great variety of forms which are being constantly developed must be addressed[12].

It is obviously crucial to consider the gap between those who have access to information, and develop the motivation and sense of personal responsibility that the health promoting style requires, and those who for a number of reasons do not. It is equally relevant to our discussion to ask whether it is realistic to assume that the majority of people may be properly informed (Mattelart, 2003) or using slightly different words, whether they are in a position to build skills for competent, critical learning.

Analyzing the functioning of information and communication agencies is of primary importance. Information, most often presented as scientifically reliable as well as easy to use, may be misleading. It is crucial to ask how such conditions relate to the perspective of a learning-based society: not only whose criteria and interests play a role in the process of knowledge formation and in patterns of communication but, perhaps more important, when and how the system makes room for -or vice versa silences-specific issues; in other words, to detect strategies of admittance into, or exclusion from, the policy-making agenda and public discourse.

Let us briefly dwell on some data. A variety of sources from sociological research and surveys, (for example, the U.N. Human Development Report, 1999) suggest that, though the general public is neither well aware nor deeply interested in scientific information in general, communication related to health appears to have the foremost relevance in whatever information and competence they show in their answers. Demand and supply of communication concerning health have been growing at an extraordinary pace. Findings from evaluation campaigns from health agencies are disseminated through widely-read journals and magazines.

This issue has been repeatedly addressed in the debate which has come to be known as "Public Understanding of Science" (1985; also Guizzardi, 2002). It has been shown on countless occasions that the media have become the most important source of health information and learning, and have the greatest impact on public opinion in practices related to health (Eurobarometer, 2000; Borgna, 2001).

Health information is channeled through an extremely well-organized system and it reaches and influences great numbers of people in their daily lives, actually, many different "audiences", or "targets", with multiple strategies: selective communication, reassurance and promotion (of products, lifestyles, symbols). The national as well as the local press, dailies and periodicals, media addressing both specialized audiences and the general public; special TV and radio programs and the internet provide medical and health information.

---

[12] A large array of research material and policy documents are available on mechanisms of communication in modern societies, in particular describing the power, influence, and overt manipulation practices of the media system. Bourdieu, with many others, focuses on the profit motive which, he says, is the primary element influencing scientific research; through the "all-powerful media apparatus" (Bourdieu 2002) advertising and marketing impact upon the political agenda-making and policy decisions.

In fact it sounds naïve to many critics to consider a self-reflexive, problematic, critical dimension of learning at all possible in the context of the continuous flow of communication, advertising and marketing and the plurality of mechanisms of information. "Alternative" sources, "underground messages", images and metaphors shape beliefs and practices both in the public and in the private sphere and impact on patterns of consumption.

The "star system" has come to play an unprecedented role in the health field (and in science in general): practitioners and scientists, patients and ex-patients, leading figures in all sorts of associations and foundations share and convey and promote information and communication. Successful people in sports and show business are also given a highly visible role.

The political as well as the theoretical relevance of this question is obvious. It focuses upon societal processes which are central to the contemporary debate: access to information and knowledge, for whom, under what conditions, hence, the unequal distribution of resources for competence, responsibility and social capabilities in everyday life; the functioning of the scientific community as it relates to political and economic institutions; in other words, issues of power and democracy.

It is within such a context that the role of health promotion and its relevance to policy-making and communication ought to be seen: not just one of the many available sources of information and health competence, we argue here, but a system of information and learning whose legitimacy is grounded on a thorough understanding of all relevant structures and processes.

I shall now briefly turn to issues of inequality and complexity because of their utmost relevance, though they are more adequately discussed in other chapters. Clearly a number of traits of the overall social organization appear to counter competent choices as far as health is concerned. Putting it bluntly: health literacy and adequate health information do not as such lead to healthy choices and living practices. There are conditions in the structure and culture of our societies which contradict assumptions of linear causality. The do-ability of health requires appropriate analysis in the context of our complex modernity.

Let us take one phenomenon of growing concern: the obesity epidemic, and the consequences of obesity-related health problems, primarily diabetes but also heart diseases and certain forms of cancer. I choose here to focus on a number of social and economic mechanisms leaving aside specifically medical problems.

Several aspects of people's everyday life need to be mentioned such as prevailing working-time patterns and conditions of urban living, which mean that many have highly demanding time-schedules. Also because of urban sprawl and suburban life people walk less than at almost any point in time, (they neither walk to work or to school, nor to do their shopping), which reduces their chances to remain active and stay fit. In many parts of the world fresh fruits and vegetables are more expensive than meat or fats of various kinds, or it may be more difficult to include them into a regular diet. Eating arrangements such as "snacking" take the place of family meals. Fast food facilities, low-priced packaged foods, the ubiquity of junk food, the availability of soda and candy even in schools are increasingly part of the everyday life experience[13]. New technological and marketing arrangements (portion sizes, vending-machines) now made available, involve growing numbers of people, the most discussed and controversial "case" being McDonald's[14].

At the global level migration from poor rural settings to city living, which is the experience of millions, entails changes that have been described as a "nutrition transition"[15]. The International Obesity Task Force 2003 Report includes data for Brazil, South Africa and China and the "transitional countries". These changes also affect other aspects in everyday experiences and lifestyles. More people become sedentary workers, more women and children live in small spaces, with no access to out of doors activities (which in many cases would mean experiencing the negative effects of highly polluted air), most likely watching television and videos.

It is also a fact that the diffusion of "global" lifestyles is in many ways enhanced because they are offered and promoted throughout the world as symbols of "western" affluence and well-being. Overall circumstances of daily life impact upon chances of leading a healthy life and the possibility of making appropriate choices.

A partly different example also pointing to elements of complexity is smoking. Worldwide campaigns aimed at measures of control on tobacco production, marketing, and use are being waged. Such measures appear however to follow a linear, somewhat simplistic, cause-effect model. One has to acknowledge that a great variety of life conditions impact upon individual or group choices. Lifestyles as adopted in youth subcultures and stressful occupational conditions, to mention two obviously different variables, counteract top-down warnings and messages about risks connected to smoking. There are in fact settings and social groups in which shared cultural models and lifestyles make smoking and alcohol drinking acceptable, even positive practices.

One last example. Worldwide statistics concerning road accidents witness the dramatically high incidence of victims, those who die as well as the even higher numbers of those who survive carrying disabilities and handicaps. Most of these victims are young men; the tragic human costs and long-lasting consequences for their life projects, as well as the financial burden for the whole society have become a significant component of the public health agenda in many countries.

Promoting education campaigns and improving safety measures (prohibiting consumption of alcohol and drugs, advising safe procedures while driving, improvement of safety equipments, and so on) are part of packages of increasingly sophisticated policies. It is evident however that especially among the youth values

---

[13] To give one figure, 15% of U.S. children are overweight: the reason: fattening food, no exercise, hours in front of TVs, computers and videogames; for adolescents, a dominant activity is "messaging".

[14] Data released by the Obesity Task Force in 2002 show that McDonald's growth, between 1996 and 2001, is set at 8% in the U.S., 23% in Canada, 76% in Europe and in Asia/Pacific/Middle East, Africa, 126%. This is also true in western societies and recently WHO has proposed a "fat tax" on junk food and limits on vending machines in schools.

[15] See United Nations, 2002.

of competitiveness and risk-taking, often taken to be positive traits of "masculinity", operate in terms of cultural and emotional rather than rational processes.

These are just some examples of the complex social processes that need to be taken into account. Conceptual frameworks and data made available in social science research no doubt add to the do-ability of health-promoting projects.

One underlying theme in all this discussion, obviously enough, is the unequal distribution of material and cultural resources in our societies, acknowledging the deep-reaching consequences, particularly in the health field, of this factor. Permanent or rather worsening inequalities at the global level, whose tragic consequences for millions in the less developed and poor parts of the world are known to all, also occur, in partly different terms, in western/ "affluent" societies. Material resources of course; but also the "cultural capital" dimension and its consequences for the learning experience are to be seen as dramatically significant for the functioning of the social system. The power dimension, public discourse and the political agenda all play a major role.

Health and wellness are to be seen within the context of profit-making and market mechanisms. Many analyses of prevailing trends in public health policies point to aspects of "commercialization", "marketization", "corporatization" (Global Social Policy, December 2002). Global business strategies and powerful private interests (in particular multinational enterprises and their apparatus of persuasion and manipulation) no doubt play a major role in the contemporary economic and political system. Intergovernmental agencies and social movements whose concerns are to reduce inequality and discrimination ceaselessly advocate that questions of health be urgently addressed in the perspective of social justice at the world level[16]. Highly dramatic figures on the distribution of wealth (hence on poverty, denied access to social services, unacceptable living conditions) are presented in international documents and debates.

In the specificity of the health promotion discourse the lack of international commitment and the utterly inadequate policies of governments and international agencies cannot be ignored. As Ilona Kickbush bluntly puts it, we witness "a form of collective amnesia" (Kickbusch, 2004). And she adds: we need" a new global social contract on health".

Considering the dimensions of power, profit-making, inequality as well as the relevance of cultural traits and personal attitudes in our highly complex societies clearly sets the present health promotion agenda within the context of modernity, both in its "enabling aspects" and in its "constraints". In the perspective of developing a health-promotion platform of policy and debate all dimensions need to be addressed as a background to the functioning of health.

As a conclusion let me just say that this is what, drawing on Pierre Bourdieu, I wanted to try and put forward: the challenge of thinking health promotion, as a scientific practice and theory, *sociologically*.

---

[16] Most recently, the Report issued by the World Commission on the Social Dimension of Globalization, A Fair Globalization: Creating Opportunities for All, ILO, 2-3-2004.

References

Abel, T., & Braun, E. (2003). Health Literacy. Wissensbasierte Gesundheitskompe-tenz; *Leitbegriffe der Gesundheitsforderung, glossar zu Konzepten, Strategien und Methoden in der Gesundheitsforderung,* BzgA, Bundeszentrale fur gesundheitliche Aufklarung.

Balbo, L. (2000). On patterns of reflexivity and lifelong learning in modern society. In B. Dausien et al. (Ed.), *Migrations-geschichten von Frauen.* Universitat Bremen.

Balbo, L. (2004). *Making a European quilt: Doing gender in the European social sciences.* Florence: European University Institute.

Bateson, G. (1972). *Steps to an ecology of mind.* New York: Ballantine.

Bateson, M.C. (1995). *Peripheral visions: Learning along the way.* New York: Harper-Collins.

Bauman Z. (1998). *Globalization: The human consequences (Themes for the 21st Century).* Oxford Cambridge: Polity Press.

Bauman, Z. (2000). *Liquid modernity,* Oxford Cambridge: Polity Press.

Beck, U. (1997). *Politik der globalisierung.* Frankfurt a. M.: Suhrkamp Verlag.

Beck, U. (1992/2000). *Risk society: Towards a new modernity (theory, culture and society series).* London: Sage Publications.

Beck, U., Giddens, A., & Lash, S. (1994). *Reflexive modernization, politics, tradition and aesthetics in the modern social order.* Stanford: Stanford University Press.

Beck, U., & Sennet R. (2000). Interview by Christiane Grefe, *Die Zeit,* April 6, 2000.

Borgna, P. (2001). *Immagini pubbliche della scienza,* Torino: Comunità.

Bourdieu, P. (1997). *Les usages sociaux de la science.* Paris: INREA.

Bourdieu, P. (2001). *Science de la Science et Reflexivité.* Paris: Raisons d'Agir.

Breslow, L. (1999). From disease prevention to health promotion. *JAMA, 281,* 1030–1033.

Castells, M. (2002). The construction of european identity. In Maria Joao Rodriguez (Ed.), *The new knowledge economy in Europe, A strategy for international competitiveness and social cohesion.* UK: MPG Books.

Commissariat au Plan. (1993). *Santé 2010. Santé, maladies et technologies.* Paris: La Documentation Française.

Davant, J.-P., Tursz, T., & Vallancien, G. (2003). *Révolution medicale.* Paris: Seuil.

Deacon, B., Ollila, E., & Stubbs, P. (2003). *Global social governance. themes and prospects.* Finland: Ministry for Social Affairs.

Durant, J., Evans, G., & Thomas, G. (1992). Public understanding of science in Britain: The role of medicine in the popular representation of science. *Public Understanding of science, 1,* 161–182.

European Commission. (1995). *White paper on teaching and learning: Towards the learning Society.* Bruxelles.

European Commission (1996). *Green paper on living and working in the information society: People first.* Bruxelles.

Giddens, A. (1990). *The consequences of modernity.* Stanford: Stanford University Press.

Giddens, A. (1991). *Modernity and self-identity. Self and society in the late modern age.* Stanford: Stanford University Press.

Gorz, A. (2003). *L' immateriel. Connaisance, valeur et capital.* Paris: Ed. Galilée.

Guizzardi, G. (Ed.). (2002). *La scienza negoziata. Scienze Biomediche nello Spazio Pubblico.* Bologna: il Mulino.

Heelas, P., Lash, S., & Morris, P. (Eds.). (1996). *Detraditionalization.* Oxford: Blackwell.

INRA-ECOSA. (2000). *The Europeans and Biotechnology: Eurobarometer 52.1.* Directorate General for Research. Directorate B—Quality of Life and Management of Living Resources. http://europa.eu.int/comm/research/pdf/eurobarometer-en.pdf

Jacobs, J. (2004). *Dark age ahead.* New York: Random House.

Kickbusch, I. (2002). Perspectives on health governance in the 20th century. In M. Marinker (Ed.), *Health Targets in Europe: Polity, progress and promise.* London: BMJ Books.

Kickbusch, I. (2004). The end of public health as we know it: Constructing global health in the 21st century. World Federation of Public Health Association Conference, The Brighton Center. Brighton, UK.

Lakoff, G. (2004). *Don't think of an elephant! know your values and frame the debate.* White River Junction, Vermont: Chelsea Green Publishing.

Lallement, M. (2003). *Temps, travail et modes de vie.* Paris: Presses Universitaires de France.

Martuccelli, D. (1999). *Sociologies de la modernité. L'itinéraire du XX siècl.* Paris: Gallimard.

Mattelart, A. (2003). *Histoire de la société de l'information.* Paris: La Decouverte.

Melucci, A. (1996). *The playing self: Person and meaning in the planetary society.* Cambridge: Cambridge University Press.

Morin, E. (1999). *Les sept savoirs nécessaires à l'éducation du futur.* Paris: UNESCO.

OECD. (2001). *The well-being of nations: The role of human and social capital.*

Popli, R. (1999). Scientific literature for all citizens. Different concepts and contexts. *Public Understanding of Science, 8*(2), 123–137.

Royal Society. (1985). *The public understanding of science.* London.

Sue, R. (2003). *La Société Civile Face au Pouvoir.* Paris: Presses de Sciences Po.

Touraine, A., & Fayard, K. (2000). *La recherche de so.* Paris: Fayard.

United Nations. (2002). *World urbanization prospects: The 2002 revision.* New York, NY: UN.

World Health Organization, Geneva. (2001). Rapport sur les médecine parallele/naturelle. *European Health Report 2000.* Copenhagen: WHO, European Regional Office.

World Commission on the Social Dimension of Globalization. (2004). *A fair globalization: Creating opportunities for all.* Geneva, Switzerland: International Labour Office.

9
Health Governance: The Health Society

Ilona Kickbusch

1. Introduction

Health and disease have physical realities, but they are also social constructs that are continuously redefined and lead to changing forms of health governance. The changing nature of health is related to and builds upon other contemporary societal trends of modernity such as individualization, differentiation, and globalization; it also contributes significantly to the concrete manifestation of these critical components of modern life. This means that health, as we understand it and live it today, is not only an outcome of other social and economic developments but a significant defining factor. The most obvious example is the increased health and life expectancy in modern societies which is redefining nearly every arena of social life and policy. Due to a lack of theory in health promotion we have not yet analyzed sufficiently how integral health is to Western modernity and who we are today.

This chapter will trace some of the developments that have made health central to modern societies and have led to the development of health promotion as a new form of health governance. It makes use of a range of sociological and historical studies with a clear bias towards the understanding of modernity as developed by Anthony Giddens (1990) and Ulrich Beck (1992).

Modernity in this understanding encompasses a long time period starting with the European enlightenment through to the present. The development of modernity is not one grand narrative, even though it is helpful to distinguish as some authors do—such as Beck (1992) and Baumann (2000)—between specific phases within it. Even these authors, however, underline that modernity is an uneven development which is characterized by its discontinuities and its double-edged character. While some authors like Bauman maintain that we have reached the end of modernity and are now in a period of post-modernity, I concur with Giddens who takes the view that we are presently moving into a period of late modernity "in which the consequences of modernity are becoming more radicalized and universalised than ever before." (1990) Following the period of the industrial revolution—which Beck calls simple modernity—we now experience the consequences and new risks of the human-constructed technological and social development that have followed in its wake.

Modernity has brought with it both vastly increased opportunities and vastly increased risks, great leaps in social development on the one hand and brutal total-itarian regimes on the other (Mazower, 1999). Giddens (1992) describes the key features of these discontinuities as being: the speed of change, the scope of change and the abstract nature of modern institutions. He also makes clear that moder-nity is inherently globalizing and produces new forms of interdependence. This "global risk society" (Beck, 1992) poses new challenges to governance and shows the limits of governing structures that were developed to answer the problems of industrialization. It also replaces the industrial notion of control and discipline with the late modern notion of flexibility and reinvention of self, (Sennet, 1998).

Modernity is highly dynamic and it has one big message: expansion. By defi-nition modernity sees itself as infinite: more is always possible, something else is always possible, there is a multiplicity of choices in everyday live. This drives the continuous increase of options, the increased participation in these options and the extension of rights to minimal participation in the options that are available. Inher-ent in the notion of expansion is the premise of progress: more is better, (Gross, 1994).

An important dimension of the debate on modernity is the manifestation of risk and choice in everyday life—indeed much of the political agenda in the risk society is set by social groups and their perception and definition of risk as well as their understanding of identity, (Giddens, 1991). Since the risk society is also a knowledge society with wide access to media and information, agendas are frequently set in the social rather than the political sphere. Beck calls this "sub-political activity": every problem of everyday life can be transformed into a political issue and a wide range of groups not involved in the "normal" political process, set agendas related to their lifestyles and "lifeworlds", (Giddens, 1998). As a consequence a "reinvention of politics" takes place. It creates a new political space with an ever increasing cast of social actors setting new themes driven by "reflexive modernization"—that is self-confrontation with the effects of risk society.

It is in such a way that individualization and differentiation not only lead to fragmentation—the patch work society or the patchwork personality—but also bring together like minded actors based on a wide variety of social definitions—women, gays, patients, persons with disabilities, environmentalists, anti globaliza-tion activists. They act for their interests beyond their relationship with economic activity in terms of class identity and classic ideological party politics of simple modernity. Giddens calls this life politics: "Life politics concern political issues which flow from processes of self actualization in post-traditional contexts, where globalising influences intrude deeply into the reflexive projects of the self, and con-versely, where processes of self-realisation influence global strategiesM (Giddens, 1991, 214).

Within modernity health has taken on a new meaning and has become a major driving force in society. Health has shaped the nature of the modern nation state and its social institutions, (Porter, 1994), it has powered social movements, defined rights of citizenship, it has contributed to the construction of the modern self and its aspirations. This chapter will attempt to describe some components of the changing nature of health by introducing the concept of the "health society". The dynamics and discontinuities in health today are generated through the interaction of three expansion processes: do-ability, territory and reflexivity.

2. The Beginning: The Enlightenment

Health is integral to the new *"modes of social life or organization which emerged in Europe from about the 17th century onwards and which subsequently became more or less worldwide in their influence"* (Giddens, 1990, 1). The creation of the health society of the 21st century has been a process long in the making and this short chapter can only highlight some of the key dimensions and turning points. To some extent the four domains of what we call the health system—personal health, public health, medical health and the health market—also represent the historical sequence of the dynamics that lead to the health society. While the systems of personal health and public health dominated the 18th and 19th centuries, during the 2oth century the medical health system gained increasing strength both in terms of its power of definition over the social construction of health and the dominance of its governance structures. It is specific to the health society that all four domains of the health system continue more or less to expand but there is a growing dominance of the market and a newly defined role of the citizen in health.

From the very beginning, the modern health discourse was characterized by the simultaneous upheaval in two spheres of life: the public and the private, the political and the personal. Health as a major new driving force shapes the state, society and politics through the creation of new social institutions and organizations while at the same time it changes the most intimate dimensions of personal and daily life. Michel Foucault stated categorically that the modern (sic) body is a "product of governance", which he analyzes primarily as a process of increased medicalization and control (Foucault, 1994). In order to fully understand the nature of the health society under conditions of late modernity it is necessary to shift this perspective to one that understands the body—and by extension health—as a core part of the construction of modern self identity and reflexivity.

With the enlightenment came the vision of being able to achieve perfect health and freedom from disease as a result of both rational science and social progress. The articles on *hygiene* and *health* by Diderot and d'Alembert in the Encyclopedie of 1776 (Sarasin, 2001) sound the beginning of the new age of reason. Disease is transformed from fate to risk: like nature disease can and must be conquered, tamed and civilized. The European enlightenment freed health from religion but linked it to morality, to the extent that health took the place of redemption. Physical health and moral health were considered to be closely interrelated and frequently the attempt to make people healthier was the entry point to make them morally better. Health was understood as the most perfect expression of the human condition, not only in the physical but in the metaphysical sense. To this day this utopian quality is reflected in many definitions of health, the most prominent being the definition adopted by the World Health Organization and included in its

Constitution: *"Health is a state of complete physical, mental and social well being, and not merely the absence of disease"* (WHO, 1948). Access to health and later to medical care became a synonym for social progress, social justice and in a historical breakthrough, the right to health was codified as a human right in the Declaration of Human Rights in 1948.

This link between health, science, governance and progress has served many ideologies, the most dangerous being those that set health as an ultimate value and combined the goal of health and of a society free of disease with totalitarian concepts of the perfect society and the perfect human being (Mazower 1998). Yet in principle the promise of health and freedom from disease through good governance combined with the application of medical and scientific discovery was achieved to an extraordinary extent and with remarkable speed in European societies. Within a very short historical time span—about 100 years—a long and more or less healthy life has become a demographic fact and a popular expectation. This success of health is in turn a driving force for many other policy developments and personal and social expectations in the health society. Indeed the very success of health creates new problems and ambiguities.

3. The Modern Governance of Health

It is one of the characteristics of the health society that **the do-ability of health** has expanded far beyond the ever rising expectations of the curative medical care and repair system. Health is considered a right and its do-ability is driven not only by universal access to the medical health system but also by the salutogenic (Antonovsky 1987) promise that *health* can be created, managed and produced by addressing the determinants of health as well as by influencing behavior and lifestyles. *More health is always possible.* Health governance in late modernity follows a conceptualization of health as "well being beyond the absence of disease" as defined by the World Health Organization in its constitution; health is linked to the capabilities and resources of individuals, communities and for society as a whole. This infinite nature of health has consequences for all four domains of the health system: it opens up new manifestations, such as wellness, and allows for the growth of a health market which attaches the added value "health" to an ever growing set of products and services. Additionally, it systematically expands the role of the state in health through new types of regulations which influence the behavior of individuals and their role in the production of health.

A modern nation state is usually seen to fulfill a number of essential functions for its members: security, rule of law, welfare and physical well being and common identity. Systems of government incorporate two principle elements: the basic institutions of governance and the organizations of governance. In governance theory, institutions are defined as the rules, norms and principles along which governance occurs and *"which define the meaning and identity of the actors and the patterns of appropriate economic, political and cultural activity engaged in by those individuals"*. In short institutions are the rules of the game. The organizations of governance are the *"material entities established to administer the provisions of governance systems"*. (Young, 1997) A health governance system in consequence must be analyzed with both the institutions and the organizations of governance in mind.

Before the industrial revolution, the state's role in securing health was limited to the cordon sanitaire and the quarantine. This was used as an attempt to defend against disease transmission and major outbreaks in order to ensure security and trade. Beyond these measures, the only existing organization of health governance, more of less, was the charitable hospital for the poor, an institution that every citizen aimed to avoid, and "bedside medicine" which was accessible for those that were better off. With the 18th century comes a revolutionary break with the past and the development of a new approach to health governance that moves it beyond security to the others functions of the modern state and the modern citizen. In their Encyclopédie Diderot and d'Alembert in 1776 (Sarasin, 2001) address the two intersecting dimensions of health governance: the public and the private. It becomes part of the role of the state to ensure health as a common good (*l'hygiène publique*) but at the same time health becomes (as *l' hygiène privée*) part of the civic and moral duty role of the individual citizen.

In modernity health **expands its territory** to become an integral part of the rules, norms and principles of social progress and the 19th century is witness to a significant expansion of both health governance organizations and institutions. In the process of modernity health becomes part of all other governing functions. The introduction and first phase of modern health governance in Europe—or what today we call the first of sanitary public health revolution (Terris, 1985) led to improved sanitation, better housing and nutrition, improved working conditions, family planning programs, compulsory immunization, maternal and child care through an extraordinary amount of laws introduced to ensure population health: vaccination acts, sanitary laws, laws that deal with living and working conditions, laws that ensure food safety as well as laws that aim to control "vices" such as alcohol and prostitution. In his later work on bio-politics in lectures held at the College de France in 1978–1979 Foucault underlines the difference between strategies developed to ensure security within everyday life and those that discipline everyday life (Foucault, 2004). We must also not forget that modern health governance was not introduced without conflict. Particularly the drastic measures taken by authorities on occasion of major outbreaks, such as small pox or cholera epidemics had great impact on the everyday lives and livelihoods of people and were often met with strong opposition (Bliss, 1991).

The link between health security and the nation state begins as early as 1810 as a number of countries on the European continent introduce compulsory small pox vaccination. In England in 1848 the first Public Health Act is adopted and in 1855 a permanent medical officer is appointed to advise the government. In the newly established German Reich the Iron Chancellor Bismarck uses the introduction of health insurance in 1883 as a mechanism to integrate the political opposition and shape the identity of the modern German nation state. In 1918 the new Soviet Union includes the right to health as one of the first articles in its new constitution. After the Second World War many European countries introduce universal access to medical care as part of the democratic entitlements of citizenship and a defining characteristic of the modern welfare state. Increasingly health governance is expanded to include safety, security and control measures, welfare and access to medical care rights and ensuring quality of life and citizen identity. Health is a driving force of the continuous expansion of the welfare state and the changing expectations of its citizens.

One of the characteristics of modern societies is that they establish abstract systems of expertise and governance to assess and manage risk. These systems represent a central feature of modernity: a disembedded mechanism "which removes social relations from the immediacy of context," (Giddens, 1990, 21). The first public health revolution was so successful because it was so essentially modern in its approach. It developed a totally new abstract system of understanding population based health risks which was provided by the realization that disease distribution is not random. While initially disease was seen to reside in the environment and attack individuals and society from the outside, the new science of statistics and the birth of epidemiology provided data which painstakingly mapped the causes of disease from within society.

This realization then structured the great debates about do-ability (intervention) and responsibility (territory) and drew the battle lines of the public health debate to this very day: does ill health produce poverty or does poverty produce ill-health? do we blame the victim or society? do we intervene with the individual or on the structural determinants? The debates around state intervention in the context of public health were not at all dissimilar to the debates around government intervention in "healthy lifestyles" today. While Edwin Chadwick, the great British reformer, found the key relationship to be between disease and dirt, Louis-René Villermé, the great French health statistician defined death as a social disease and outlined how medicine, guided by political economy, must and will become a social science. This view was later echoed by Rudolf Virchow and all those committed to what would be called "social medicine". What united these very different political orientations was their joint expectation that one day there would be an end point, when the battle against disease will have been won through the efforts of society. "All believed", says J.N. Hays of the great sanitarians "in the power of civilization to eradicate disease," (Hays, 1998).

This changed, as in the 20th century health governance the power to eradicate disease shifted from society and public health to medicine. The triumph of the germ theory over environmental approaches began on March 24, 1882, when Robert Koch announced that the tubercle bacillus was the cause of tuberculosis. Health became do-able in a new and, it seemed, much more efficient way. The new medical knowledge allowed the focused attack on the agent of the disease—the germ, the bacillus, the virus—rather than having to deal with a complex environment or difficult populations. As drugs and technology became increasingly available, the power to eradicate disease was seen to reside with medicine rather than with social progress, indeed the progress of medicine was equated with social progress and the sanitary and the social perspective made way for an individualistic view of health and disease, (Porter, 1997).

Yet it was the very success of the social perspective and the political public health that made the success of the medical system possible. Mortality had been reduced by an extraordinary extent in a very short period of time, (McKeown, 1980), and by the early decades of the 20th century living conditions had improved considerably and led to new social expectations. For example the high levels of maternal and infant death were no longer socially and politically acceptable, particularly to women who had gained rights of citizenship and could cast their vote. In addition European nations were suffering from the impact of the 1914–18 war and the 1918 flu epidemic. There was strong pressure on politicians to instigate measures that would provide hope for the future and bind voters and the political demand that emerged (and has remained to this day) was for more access to medicine and its promise.

It is at this point that the health governance perspective shifts radically and moves into the dominant mode of expert medical care provision—which rapidly gains more power than the by now established public health system. It also overshadows the system of self determined personal health. The term health loses its many dimensions and part of its power of emancipation and becomes synonymous with medical care. In Europe, this is achieved through an extraordinary coalition between medicine and the expanding welfare state, which begins to guarantee an increasing number of social rights. The—wrongly named—health system grows at an astonishing speed and through new financing mechanisms such as medical insurance (usually linked to the workplace) increasing numbers of the population gain access. European countries reach near universal coverage by the mid 20th century, and medical and technological developments, as well as demographic shifts, drive its continuous expansion. The leading health governance principle in the welfare state had paradoxically shifted from addressing the needs of population health to treating the individual citizen; in the process, it transformed the ideal of the participating and knowledgeable citizen of the enlightenment era into the passive and compliant patient who follows the physician's instruction.

4. The Expansion of the Territory of Health

Yet only fifty years later the shift towards the health society sets in. The expansion of life and health expectancy, the high level of security in welfare states, the increase in education levels and health knowledge and the democratization of society continue to drive the ever increasing expectations towards the medical system and what it can do—but they also drive individualization and increase the reflexivity about the very process. As health increases so do personal expectations of ever better health and the recognition that modern society itself has become a "risk environment" for health. The body is perennially at risk even in the most familiar surroundings (Giddens, 1990), risks lurk in food, in the air, at home, at work, in the street and the most intimate pleasures become risk behaviors. Health security threats are also consistently referred to as one of the most disturbing consequences of globalization, either as terrorist threats (for example anthrax or small pox virus) or infectious disease threats, such as the avian flu, (Chen et al. 2003).

Not only were the expectations that had been generated by the marriage of modernity and medical progress only partially fulfilled, the germ based cause effect model was also ever more difficult to apply to the health profile of late modernity which had shifted to non infectious diseases, also frequently referred to as lifestyle diseases. Initially the medical system turns to a personal health model and delegates the prevention challenge into ever increasing expectations towards individuals to choose rational and responsible health behaviors The limits of such a model became clear at many levels: not only do health choices depend on many factors other than knowledge, but the equation of the enlightenment as formulated by Immanuel Kant "to know and to be certain" no longer applies under conditions of late modernity. There is always more to know and what is considered healthy today may not be healthy tomorrow as illustrated in the decade long struggle over the effects of alcohol on health.

Healthy choices are complex within a "risk society" where unknown and un-expected risks emerge over which the individual has no control whatsoever and which are a consequence of progress itself, such as environmental risks. Or where old risks are communicated in new ways and are suddenly in the center of attention, such as certain rules of nutrition. The most intimate actions—such as nursing a child or having sex with strangers—are connected to distant outbreaks (such as the events of Tschernobyl or the advent of HIV/AIDS) and are subject to new knowl-edge and revisions of behavior. They constantly alter their character, (Giddens, 1990, 38), and in contradictory turnabouts the breast is not always best and sexual adventures need to be practiced as "safe sex".

The risk profile of late modernity emplies that solutions need to be found beyond the medical health system and that health policy needs to concern itself with investments in other parts of society. Finally the growth of the medical health system itself begins to be seen as counterproductive: "A society that spends so much on health care that it cannot or will not spend adequately on other health enhancing activities may actually be reducing the health of its population." (Evans & Stoddard, 1994).

The massive health education campaigns that were conducted in this period alter both the perception and the experience of health risk and support an increasing awareness of limitations of medical expertise and the application of the cause effect model. Health moves out of the expert medical system into the context of everyday life and everyday behavior and becomes ever more open to social rather then medical definitions and constructions. This drives the **expansion of the territory of health.** *Health is everywhere.* It is created—to quote the Ottawa Charter for Health Promotion, the seminal WHO document that originated in 1986—"where people live, love, work and play". (WHO, 1986)

A broad understanding of health determinants beyond the classic determinants of income and poverty—ranging from social support to the hierarchical structures of society, from gender to race, the organization of work to the social cohesion and social capital of communities—not only expands the health policy arena into wide range of other sectors but also expand its policy reach into the most intimate areas of personal life and behavior.(Blane et al, 1996) These health determinants are complex and do not respond to simple cause and effect models, they are frequently not visible, build up over long time periods and usually need a cluster of responses and interventions that present policy and administrative structures do not allow.

The contradictions inherent to the health society and its expansions make health a prominent feature in social and political discourse. Modernity's promise of universality and inclusive citizenship and its reality of systemic exclusion (Breman, 2004) are perhaps more tangible in health than in other policy arenas. An ever increasing array of health actors participate in the shaping of a 21st century understanding of health and its role for the individual and for society. A major expression is the rise of identity politics in health, through which groups which define themselves through a common health claim or disease characteristic come together as political actors to demand more recognition, more prevention, more research or more services. The dominant issue at stake is no longer "medicalization" and the power of the medical profession, rather the debate evolves around privatization and commercialization, empowerment and participation, social inclusion and exclusion, public and private.

This is exemplified through the wellness revolution which marries personal health and the market, choice and do-ability. Health translates into a product that can be bought on the market, promises wellbeing and changes the citizen into a consumer. Health is considered "the next big thing of the 21st century .... which promises to revolutionize our lives and offers opportunities for tremendous wealth building over the next ten years". (Pilzer, 2002) These health goods and services include the fitness market, cosmetic surgery, lifestyle drugs such as Viagra and the market for vitamins, minerals and health foods. They also include new types of health insurance, which would pay for health not sickness services and which would reimburse the tools and services the new industry has to offer. Calculations indicate that in the United States alone the sales of the wellness industry have already reached approximately $200 billion and that it is set to achieve sales of $ 1 trillion within 10 years. For many existing industries health has become an "active added value" either as a sales pitch or in the form of supplements and product enhancements. Providing access to information on health and new health products and services including e-health becomes one of the greatest business opportunities of the foreseeable future. In the typical ambiguity of developments under modernity the market also provides the opportunity for consumer movements to engage for products and services that create health.

But the danger of widening the health gap grows, as the healthy and better off buy an ever increasing amount of health and wellness while cuts in the public sector not only reduce prevention and health education services for the poor (for example nutrition education) but also weaken public safeguards on harmful goods and services (for example access to and advertising of soft drinks and junk food in US schools).

5. The Expansion of Reflexivity of Health

As do-ability increases so do options, choices and insecurity. *Every choice in daily life potentially becomes a choice for or against health*. This leads to the

expansion of the reflexivity of health. The revolutionary change and promise of health governance that came with the European enlightenment of the 18th century was that health is not a natural state but can be produced and created through the application of scientific progress and knowledge once the will and the commitment to act is generated. Science would provide the basis for rational governance for the common good. But as one of the consequences of modernity this belief in rationality has been shattered: many of the health risks are linked to the development of modernity itself and frequently science—despite its infinite promise of genetics and biotechnology—has no answers for common health problems in everyday life.

At this point of modernity knowledge no longer means certitude. As the risks are frequently not visible and intangible they need to be communicated and above all understood and translated into action. As more and new health information becomes available health practices need to be constantly revisited and revised, a constant reappraisal of actions under conditions of uncertainty, both by policy makers and ordinary citizens is necessary. The expansion of health choices demands an ever higher degree of sophistication, participation and literacy and in consequence there is a growing offer and demand for health information.

With the introduction of public health as a function of the modern state, health moves from a personal ideal of the individual citoyen and man of means to a concern of the emerging working class as well as the larger population. Sarasin provides a nice wordplay on the changes between the 18th and the 19th century conception of personal health: in the 18th century the emancipated citoyen, a member of an exclusive group, needed to know everything about his body, now in the mid 19th century everybody needs to know about health. (Sarasin, 2001, p. 120) This could only be achieved though a major educational effort and democratization of health knowledge and we witness the beginning of the age of mass hygiene education.

Health provides a sense of purpose to a wide range of philanthropic and political societies who saw it as their ultimate goal to improve the health knowledge (and frequently the morals) of the working classes and the excluded members of society. What had been true for the citoyen—empowerment and emancipation through health—now was presented as a message for everybody in a flood of journals, books, lectures and pamphlets—but also as part of political mobilization. For example in 1895 191 journals were published on Paris in the field of medicine and hygiene—21 were for general readers and the most popular was the Journal de la Santé with 29 000 subscribers. (Sarasin, 2001)

But health also forms part of political mobilization and moves into the realm of rights and of equity. Indeed from the 19th century on claims for access to health and access to citizenship increasingly converge and become a driving force of social and political movements while opponents decry the increasing influence of the state on the individual and his health decisions. Walter Holland quotes a Leader in *The Times (1854) which states: "we prefer to take our chance of cholera and the rest than be bullied into health"*. (Holland & Stewart, 1998) Yet by the early 20th century the role of the modern state in health governance was firmly established through public health systems and social reformers and conservative politicians, radical social movements, professional societies, philanthropies, civil society and the market, all participate in the attempt to define and order the territory of health. Health governance is always about inclusion and exclusion and health governance debates are always also about social justice. Health became part of the political agenda because increasingly all parts of society understood that health was do-able and early death and disease were accepted less and less. A consensus began to emerge that through public health measures society had a responsibility to address health inequalities and protect the population's health.

The citizen/citoyen that Diderot and d'Álembert had in mind was a man. De-nial of equal citizenship to women was—as widely documented in the feminist literature—paralleled by the denial of having control over their own bodies, their sexuality and their reproductive capacity. It was the male body that entered the public sphere and that became the norm for what it meant to be healthy. To be female was to be the other, the private, the non-citizen. In consequence the early feminists who fought for the right to vote argued that their bodies (as bearers of children) were as important to the state as the male body (as a soldier defending the nation). Women's health has remained an exemplary area of the interface between health rights and civil, political and social rights to this day. The women's health movement of the 1960ies and 70ies makes personal health into a political program exemplified in slogans such as "the personal is political" or "my body belongs to me". And most recently through the AIDS movements of the 80ies and 90ies health has become a social and political force of integration and access first for the excluded gay community then for the excluded poor in developing countries. The present global drive for access to AIDS medicines for developing nations is the spearhead of a global citizenship movement.

6. Health Promotion: A New Health Governance Map

The development of the health society is part of a general change in social values (Inglehardt, 2000) linked to modernity which are usually described with the fol-lowing characteristics: Individualization, Differentiation, recognition of the value of autonomy and self-responsibility, subjective/holistic well being, high expecta-tions and quality of life. These social trends correspond with the epidemiological development symbolized by the two public health revolutions that changed the face of health and disease in the 19th and 20th century. The major improvements in living conditions and health make major shifts in the overall organization of modern societies possible. The citizens become participants in health creation and health decision-making with all the ambivalence it implies: the continuous pro-cesses of individualization have widened choices and life options (empowerment) but have also led to an increased delegation of risk management to the individual, the family the community. (Lupton, 1999)

A new governance map for health was drawn in the 1970ies with the publication of two seminal reports. The first "A new perspective on the health of Canadians" was developed in 1974 under the responsibility of health minister Marc Lalonde (Lalonde, 1974) and presented a health field concept which was to significantly influence the health policy approach of many OECD countries for years to come, in particular when used by the WHO as a model for its own policy approach. The second was "Our Bodies—Ourselves" by The Boston Women's Health Collective, a book "by and for women" which shattered all views held so far of women's health and heralded a new level of involvement of people in defining and creating their own health (The Boston Women's Health Collective, 1970). Together they laid the strategic foundations for the third public health revolution and health promotion.

The Lalonde report stated that in order to achieve better population health— or to stay in the terminology of this chapter to address the health risks of late modernity—four fields of determinants must be addressed: biological factors, the physical and social environment, lifestyle factors and health care services. The report highlighted that many if not most of the factors determining population health were outside of the remit of the health services and initiated a new phase of the expansion of the territory of health, which in turn was to nurture the WHO Ottawa Charter on Health Promotion. (WHO, 1986) This charter reframed the Lalonde domains as: healthy public policy, supportive environments, community action, personal skills and reoriented health care systems. The Lalonde Report as well as the Ottawa Charter showed clearly that health care services were only part of the solution; indeed they might also be part of the problem and needed to change radically.

The seventies and eighties saw the ascent of two strategic approaches which tried to move health away from the medical model of production and control. One was through the introduction of technocratic strategies from the private sector into the health arena as exemplified by the US Health Objectives for the Nation which introduced an approach to plan for health by setting measurable goals and targets. (US Public Health Service, 1979) The movement to construct health targets was an attempt to govern the expansion of territory and risk in modern society through professional strategies. In contrast "Our Bodies—Ourselves" by The Boston Women's Health Collective, sounded the start for a new type of citizens involvement for the power of definition in health and showed that many of the issues that were defined as biological differences by science and the medical profession as being social and political. It was the women's health movement that most clearly expressed the direction health was to take at the end of the 20th century as individualization and identity politics become political program: the personal is political and my body belongs to me. This was echoed—albeit in less radical form—in the growth of the self help movement and the many patient organizations where citizens set out to become experts in their own disease. (Kickbusch, 2002a)

Analyzing the Ottawa Charter for Health Promotion through the analytical constructs of modernity theory and the health society shows the extent to which it responded to all three expansion dynamics of the health society. Its success can probably be explained by the fact that it is the first health policy document to fully reflect and codify the role of health in late modernity, an approach that is often referred to as "the new public health". It defined health to be a resource and an integral part of everyday life, it acknowledged and legitimized the expansion of the territory of health and proposed policy actions in all sectors of society through "healthy public policy", It based its proposals on the salutogenic promise that health is doable: it can be created but at the same time it made clear that this creation involved the citizens and the communities themselves in a participatory process. The definition of health promotion first and foremost recognizes people as social actors and agents and has a focus on their empowerment in the sense of lifepolitics: health promotion is the process to increase control of people over their health.

In consequences some authors (for example Petersen, 1996) contend that this is not a move towards empowerment but an increased privatization of risk. Yet this is much too narrow an interpretation rooted in the control and discipline paradigm, rather than in the paradigm of reflexive modernity. The Charter reflects the ambiguous "fit" with wider social trends under way that define and structure everyday life. We can now—in the words of Lester Breslow, (1999) a leading social epidemiologist—"turn more attention to the nature of health and regard it ... as a resource for living" and we can focus health promotion strategies on "capacity building for health". He terms this the third public health revolution. Within this revolution *l'hygiène publique and l'hygiene privée* are both necessary and legitimate and intertwined in a wide variety of ways.

A shift to a model of health promotion recognizes the importance of the structural dimensions of a public health approach to health governance as put astutely by Rose (1992): "*the primary determinants of disease are mainly economic and social, therefore its remedies must also be economic and social.*" Yet it assigns a much large role to citizens as social actors in all four domains of the health system. Its premise is that despite all ambiguities social change for health is possible and that systems can be changed through radical engagement and collective action. It is because of this empowerment dimension that health promotion is more than a professional strategy and why frequently it has taken on the character of a social movement. Health promotion reinterprets the message of The Boston Women's Health Collective in the form of modern life politics: the choices we make in health everyday are indeed not just about our weight or our smoking habits; they are political in their own right and have political consequences not only of a local but of a global nature. The litigation cases against the tobacco and the fast food companies are a case in point as is the debate around TRIPS in the World Trade Organization. They attempt—as Beck would put it—a constant day by day answer to the question *"How do we want to live?"*

7. The Deterritorialization of Health

A number of key dimensions define health in the health society.

First: the health society implies that health is present in every dimension of life. In its mirror image it also implies that risk is everywhere. This has significant consequences for how we frame health policies and where we assign responsibilities for health in society. If health is everywhere every place or setting in society can support or endanger health. Stakeholders in the big health debate are not only the producers of unhealthy products and substances but the arenas of everyday life where they are consumed. One of the consequences of the health society is a shift from material entities and organizations that are clearly defined as "health organizations" (in this case the medical care system we tend to call the health system) to an increased dependence on institutional mechanisms which apply throughout society and which regulate behaviors and the access to or the consumption of products.

Typical examples are smoking regulations: they not only regulate who can buy tobacco products, where and at what price but they also regulate where it is permitted to smoke. Over time smoking restrictions expand to all settings in society: first usually schools and hospitals, then major public places, then all forms of transport, then restaurants and bars until finally—as is the case now in New York, practically no space remains outside the home where smoking is permitted. Smoking laws also regulate the access to images and message through the restriction of advertising for tobacco products. Health it turns out really is everybody's business in a symbolic and a real sense: owners of bars and restaurants, retailers, the management of airports and railway lines to name but a few, all need to be concerned with health. Settings of everyday life become "healthy" settings through a commitment to norms and standards and patterns of appropriate behavior—with laws and regulations sometimes promoting, in other cases following cultural shifts. (Kickbusch, 2003)

Second: we are therefore not only witnessing an expansion of the territory of health—increasingly we are witness to its de-territorialization. Health policy becomes ever more virtual—it moves in a new political space with a new quality, it transcends functional specialization but is clearly subject to increased individualization and differentiation. This raises a number of issues in sociological theory in which the "health system" is frequently referred to as a subsystem which is committed to a certain functional specialization that only it can fulfill. According to Niklas Luhmann (1995) such a functional subsystem is organised around a binary code, which controls the selection of decision belonging to the subsystem. In this case the health system's reference point would be the binary reference code disease—health.

This may well apply to disease and the medical system—which Luhmann probably had in mind—but it does not apply to health. The territory of the medical system continues to grow continuously and can be relatively clearly circumscribed, the territory of health not only grows, it becomes ever less tangible. This de territorialization is of course the reason for the modern health policy paradox: *"One of the great paradoxes in the history of health policy is that, despite all the evidence and understanding that has accrued about determinants of health and the means available to tackle them, the national and international policy arenas are filled with something quite different"*. (Leppo, 1998). Policy in health societies is out of sink and still frames "health" in terms of expenditure and consumption of health care services and very few institutions, organizations and funding programs clearly differentiate between program that focus on *health* and those that focus on health care.

Third: in the health society health has become a "co-produced" good which needs the cooperation of many sectors and actors in society. Not only must the synergy of the four domains of the health system—personal health, public health, medical health and the health market—be harnessed but it is also necessary to gain the support of policy arenas such as environment, labor, agriculture and education to name but a few. Yet there are very few policy mechanisms that allow this to happen in an integrative manner. Each of the health domains in turn has its own contradictory driving forces—control/empowerment, risk/social reform, expert knowledge and profit—and has developed its own set of categories of governance of the body and the body politic. At the same time the role of the state in ensuring health security is subject to major shifts. The governance of what in most of the literature is called the "health system" (but rarely deals with health), is due for a revolutionary overhaul due to financial, technological and demographic developments.

Fourth: in the health society the salutogenic governance premise is investment related to the ubiquity of health. It proposes that the health dollar is best spent by productively reorienting it towards the production of health or, in the terminology of the third public health revolution towards resources and capabilities. The focus of health policy then is to produce a larger health gain for society, irrespective of sectoral divisions. This of course is difficult because no functional system exists within governance systems of late modern societies to respond to a deterritorialized policy arena and policy in late modern societies. This results in what has been called "organized irresponsibility". (Beck) Each policy (sub)system concentrates on it own logic and intentions without regard for the impact on other areas of society. This can only be partially and insufficiently addressed through mechanisms of health impact statements, particularly given the expansion of health in the marketplace.

Fifth: in the health society the domain of personal health returns to the fore in a new form: with increasing autonomy, individualization, and choice. Individuals do not only have an increased interest they also have increased responsibility for their own health. The expansion of rights ensures the expansion coverage and new forms of prevention, for example the rights of non smokers but it also leads to increasing fragmentation in the combination with the increasing do-ablity through medical and pharmaceutical strategies. It raises new questions of solidarity far beyond the basic questions of protection and coverage dealt with by the early health movements. Is infertility and in vitro fertilization an issue for coverage? Should there be higher premiums for people with unhealthy lifestyles?

Finally, as health increasingly drives economic and social development we need to begin to answer the political questions at stake in the health society. How do we want to define health security and health solidarity? What extent of exclusion and inequality will be politically accepted? What social, political and financial price are we willing to pay for better health both individually and as a community, both at the local and at the global level? While it seems unfair that some parts of society can buy better health in the marketplace—where do we see the limits? While it seems appropriate to strive for more health should we not also critically consider the limits of this quest? These questions cannot be resolved without a debate on the values which will ultimately drive the health society.

As a consequence of the three expansions the health society carries within it three promises of health: health as an ultimate value, health as a product on the market place or health as a project of empowerment. (Kickbusch, 2002b) F. Fukuyama (2002) in his analysis of the consequences of the biotechnology revolution highlights how it might put into question not only all our assumptions on human nature but also the underpinnings of democracy with its premise that all human beings are created equal. Z. Baumann (1989) in particular has highlighted, that there is an inherent connection between modernity and totalitarianism if the democratic component—the dimension of the citoyen—is neglected. The utopian "total" quality of the health promise of the enlightenment was balanced by the moral obligations of the citoyen as a free political actor. Throughout modernity the involvement of people in their health has offered an extraordinary emancipatory impetus and it is the strength of health promotion as codified in the Ottawa Charter that its vision of health under conditions of modernity is deeply democratic and participatory. It is the role of citizen in health—as most of the theoretical analyses of modernity would agree—that becomes the most critical component of health governance in the 21st century. A theoretical perspective can help us understand why.

References

Antonovsky, A. (1987). *Unraveling the mystery of health. How people manage stress and stay well.* San Francisco: Jossey Bass.

Bauman, Z. (1989). *Modernity and the Holocaust.* Cambridge: Polity Press.

Baumann Z. (2000). *Liquid modernity.* Cambridge: Polity Press.

Beck, U. (1992). *Risk society.* Cambridge: Polity Press.

Blane, D., Brunner, E., & Wilkinson, R. (1996). *Health and social organization.* London and New York: Routledge.

Bliss, M. (1919). *Plague—how smallpox devastated Montreal.* Toronto, Ontario: Harper-Collins.

Breman, J. (2004). *Social exclusion in the context of globalization* (Working paper No. 18). Geneva: International Labor Office.

Breslow, L. (1999). From disease prevention to health promotion. *JAMA, 281,* 1030–1033.

Chen, L., Leaning, J., & Narasimhan, V. (2003). *Global health challenges for human security.* Boston, MA: Harvard University.

Evans, R. G., & Stoddart, G. L. (1994). Producing health, consuming health care. In R. G. Evans et al. (Eds.), *Why are some people healthy and others not?* (pp. 27–64). New York: Aldine de Gruyter.

Foucault, M. (1994). *The birth of the clinic. An archaeology of medical perception.* New York: Vintage Press Random House.

Foucault, M. (2004). *Naissance de la biopolitique*. Paris: Editions Gallimard/ Editions de Seuil.

Fukuyama, F. (2002). *Our posthuman future. Consequences of the biotechnology revolution*. New York: Farrar, Straus and Giroux.

Giddens, A. (1990). *The consequences of modernity*. Stanford, CA: Stanford University Press.

Giddens, A. (1991). *Modernity and self-identity: Self and society in the late modern age*. Stanford, CA: Stanford University Press.

Gross, P. (1994). *Die Multioptionsgesellschaft*. Frankfurt am Main: Suhrkamp.

Hays, J. N. (1998). *The burdens of disease: Epidemics and human response in Western history*. New Brunswick, NJ: Rutgers University Press.

Holland, W. W., & Stewart S. (1998). *Public health: The vision and the challenge*. London: Nuffield Trust.

Inglehart, R., & Baker, W. E. (2000). Modernization, cultural change and the persistence of traditional values. *American Sociological Review*, 65(1), 19–51.

Kickbusch, I. (2002a). Perspectives on health governance in the 21st century: Revisiting health goals and targets. In: M. Marinker (Ed.), *Health Targets in Europe: Polity, Progress and Promise*. London: BMJ Books, 206–229.

Kickbusch, I. (2002b). The future value of health. Perspectives in Health. *Pan American Health Organization Magazine*, Centennial issue, 7, 28–32.

Kickbusch, I. (2003). Perspectives in health promotion and population health. *American Journal of Public Health, 93*, 383–388.

Lalonde, M. (1974). *A new perspective on the health of Canadians*. Canada: Government of Canada.

Leppo, K. (1998). Introduction. In M. Koivisalu, & E. Ollila (Eds.), *Making a healthy world*. London: Zed Books.

Luhmann, N. (1995). *Social systems*. Stanford: Stanford University Press.

Lupton, D. (Ed.). (1999). *Risk and socio cultural theory, new directions and perspectives*. Cambridge: Cambridge University Press.

Mazower, M. (1999). *Dark Continent Europe's Twentieth Century*. New York: Knopf.

McGinnis, J. M., & Foege, W. H. (1993). Actual causes of death in the United States. *JAMA*, 270, 2207–2212.

McKeown, T. (1980). *The role of medicine: Dream, mirage or nemesis*. Princeton: Princeton University Press.

Metzler, G. (2003). Der deutsche Sozialstaat. Stuttgart: Deutsche Verlagsanstalt. Vom bismarckschen Erfolgsmodell zum Pflegefall. Stuttgard/München.

Petersen, A. R. (1996). Risk and the regulated self: The discourse of health promotion as politics of uncertainty. *Australian and New Zealand Journal of Sociology*, 32, 44–57.

Pilzer, P. Z. (2002). *The wellness revolution. How to make a fortune in the next trillion dollar industry*. New York: John Wiley and Sons.

Porter, D. (Ed.). (1994). *The history of public health and the modern state*. Amsterdam: editions Rodopi.

Porter, R. (1997). *The greatest benefit to mankind*. London: HarperCollins.

Rose, G. (1992). *The strategy of preventive medicine*. Oxford: Oxford University Press.

Sarasin, P. (2001). *Reizbare Maschinen*. Frankfurt: M Suhrkamp.

Sennet, R. (1998). *The corrosion of character*. New York and London: W. W. Norton.

Terris, M. (1985). The changing relationships of epidemiology and society. *Journal of Public Health Policy, 6*, 15–36.

The Boston Women's Health Collective (1970). *Our bodies, ourselves*. Boston, MA: Simon & Schuster.

US Public Health Service. (1979). *Healthy people: Surgeon General's report on health promotion and disease prevention*. Washington, DC: Government Printing Office.

World Health Organization (WHO). (1986). Ottawa charter for health promotion. *Health Promotion, 1*, iii–v.

World Health Organization (WHO). (1948). *Constitution*.

Young, O. (Ed.). (1997). *Global governance*. Cambridge, MA: MIT press.

Appendix

Ottawa Charter for Health Promotion
First International Conference on Health Promotion
Ottawa, 21 November 1986—WHO/HPR/HEP/95.1*

The first International Conference on Health Promotion, meeting in Ottawa this 21st day of November 1986, hereby presents this CHARTER for action to achieve Health for All by the year 2000 and beyond.

This conference was primarily a response to growing expectations for a new public health movement around the world. Discussions focused on the needs in industrialized countries, but took into account similar concerns in all other regions. It built on the progress made through the Declaration on Primary Health Care at Alma-Ata, the World Health Organization's Targets for Health for All document, and the recent debate at the World Health Assembly on intersectoral action for health.

Health Promotion

Health promotion is the process of enabling people to increase control over, and to improve, their health. To reach a state of complete physical, mental and social well-being, an individual or group must be able to identify and to realize aspirations, to satisfy needs, and to change or cope with the environment. Health is, therefore, seen as a resource for everyday life, not the objective of living. Health is a positive concept emphasizing social and personal resources, as well as physical capacities. Therefore, health promotion is not just the responsibility of the health sector, but goes beyond healthy life-styles to well-being.

Prerequisites for Health

The fundamental conditions and resources for health are:

• peace

---

* Charter adopted at an international conference on health promotion: The move towards a new public health, November 17–21, 1986, Ottawa, Ontario, Canada. Co-sponsored by the Canadian Public Health Association, Health and Welfare Canada, and the World Health Organization.

- shelter
- education
- food
- income
- a stable eco-system
- sustainable resources
- social justice, and equity.

Improvement in health requires a secure foundation in these basic prerequisites.

Advocate

Good health is a major resource for social, economic and personal development and an important dimension of quality of life. Political, economic, social, cultural, environmental, behavioural and biological factors can all favour health or be harmful to it. Health promotion action aims at making these conditions favourable through advocacy for health.

Enable

Health promotion focuses on achieving equity in health. Health promotion action aims at reducing differences in current health status and ensuring equal opportunities and resources to enable all people to achieve their fullest health potential. This includes a secure foundation in a supportive environment, access to information, life skills and opportunities for making healthy choices. People cannot achieve their fullest health potential unless they are able to take control of those things which determine their health. This must apply equally to women and men.

Mediate

The prerequisites and prospects for health cannot be ensured by the health sector alone. More importantly, health promotion demands coordinated action by all concerned: by governments, by health and other social and economic sectors, by nongovernmental and voluntary organization, by local authorities, by industry and by the media. People in all walks of life are involved as individuals, families and communities. Professional and social groups and health personnel have a major responsibility to mediate between differing interests in society for the pursuit of health.

Health promotion strategies and programmes should be adapted to the local needs and possibilities of individual countries and regions to take into account differing social, cultural and economic systems.

Health Promotion Action Means

Build Healthy Public Policy

Health promotion goes beyond health care. It puts health on the agenda of policy makers in all sectors and at all levels, directing them to be aware of the health consequences of their decisions and to accept their responsibilities for health.

Health promotion policy combines diverse but complementary approaches including legislation, fiscal measures, taxation and organizational change. It is coordinated action that leads to health, income and social policies that foster greater equity. Joint action contributes to ensuring safer and healthier goods and services, healthier public services, and cleaner, more enjoyable environments.

Health promotion policy requires the identification of obstacles to the adoption of healthy public policies in non-health sectors, and ways of removing them. The aim must be to make the healthier choice the easier choice for policy makers as well.

Create Supportive Environments

Our societies are complex and interrelated. Health cannot be separated from other goals. The inextricable links between people and their environment constitutes the basis for a socioecological approach to health. The overall guiding principle for the world, nations, regions and communities alike, is the need to encourage reciprocal maintenance—to take care of each other, our communities and our natural environment. The conservation of natural resources throughout the world should be emphasized as a global responsibility.

Changing patterns of life, work and leisure have a significant impact on health. Work and leisure should be a source of health for people. The way society organizes work should help create a healthy society. Health promotion generates living and working conditions that are safe, stimulating, satisfying and enjoyable.

Systematic assessment of the health impact of a rapidly changing environment— particularly in areas of technology, work, energy production and urbanization— is essential and must be followed by action to ensure positive benefit to the health of the public. The protection of the natural and built environments and the conservation of natural resources must be addressed in any health promotion strategy.

Strengthen Community Actions

Health promotion works through concrete and effective community action in setting priorities, making decisions, planning strategies and implementing them to achieve better health. At the heart of this process is the empowerment of communities—their ownership and control of their own endeavours and destinies.

Community development draws on existing human and material resources in the community to enhance self-help and social support, and to develop flexible systems for strengthening public participation in and direction of health matters. This requires full and continuous access to information, learning opportunities for health, as well as funding support.

Develop Personal Skills

Health promotion supports personal and social development through providing information, education for health, and enhancing life skills. By so doing, it increases the options available to people to exercise more control over their own health and over their environments, and to make choices conducive to health.

Enabling people to learn, throughout life, to prepare themselves for all of its stages and to cope with chronic illness and injuries is essential. This has to be facilitated in school, home, work and community settings. Action is required through educational, professional, commercial and voluntary bodies, and within the institutions themselves.

Reorient Health Services

The responsibility for health promotion in health services is shared among individuals, community groups, health professionals, health service institutions and governments. They must work together towards a health care system which contributes to the pursuit of health.

The role of the health sector must move increasingly in a health promotion direction, beyond its responsibility for providing clinical and curative services. Health services need to embrace an expanded mandate which is sensitive and respects cultural needs. This mandate should support the needs of individuals and communities for a healthier life, and open channels between the health sector and broader social, political, economic and physical environmental components.

Reorienting health services also requires stronger attention to health research as well as changes in professional education and training. This must lead to a change of attitude and organization of health services which refocuses on the total needs of the individual as a whole person.

Moving into the Future

Health is created and lived by people within the settings of their everyday life; where they learn, work, play and love. Health is created by caring for oneself and others, by being able to take decisions and have control over one's life circumstances, and by ensuring that the society one lives in creates conditions that allow the attainment of health by all its members.

Caring, holism and ecology are essential issues in developing strategies for health promotion. Therefore, those involved should take as a guiding principle that, in each phase of planning, implementation and evaluation of health promotion activities, women and men should become equal partners.

Commitment to Health Promotion

The participants in this Conference pledge:

- to move into the arena of healthy public policy, and to advocate a clear political commitment to health and equity in all sectors;
- to counteract the pressures towards harmful products, resource depletion, unhealthy living conditions and environments, and bad nutrition; and to focus attention on public health issues such as pollution, occupational hazards, housing and settlements;
- to respond to the health gap within and between societies, and to tackle the inequities in health produced by the rules and practices of these societies;
- to acknowledge people as the main health resource; to support and enable them to keep themselves, their families and friends healthy through financial and other means; and to accept the community as the essential voice in matters of its health, living conditions and well-being;
- to reorient health services and their resources towards the promotion of health; and to share power with other sectors, other disciplines and, most importantly, with people themselves;
- to recognize health and its maintenance as a major social investment and challenge; and to address the overall ecological issue of our ways of living.

The Conference urges all concerned to join them in their commitment to a strong public health alliance.

Call for International Action

The Conference calls on the World Health Organization and other international organizations to advocate the promotion of health in all appropriate forums and to support countries in setting up strategies and programmes for health promotion.

The Conference is firmly convinced that if people in all walks of life, nongovernmental and voluntary organizations, governments, the World Health Organization and all other bodies concerned join forces in introducing strategies for health promotion, in line with the moral and social values that form the basis of this CHARTER, Health For All by the year 2000 will become a reality.

Index

170

Printed in the United States
93879LV00002BA